Critical Discourses of Old Age and Telecare Technologies

This book makes an enquiry into policies surrounding old age and telecare. It contextualises telecare within the wider history of health and social care in England to build the case that there are grand narratives of old age embedded in policies.

Divided into four sections, the book covers:

- Connecting old age with telecare
- A general review of old age and telecare
- A critical enquiry into discourses and the identity of old age
- Conclusions and future directions.

The author highlights the manifestation of old age discourses in care policies, how they have been perpetuated yet also transformed in the context of telecare, and what this means about older people. The book will be of interest to students and academics in the fields of gerontology, sociology, old age studies, philosophy, social policy, health and social care policy, information systems, and critical theoreticians.

Gizdem Akdur is a research fellow at the Centre for Research in Public Health and Community Care (CRIPACC) of the University of Hertfordshire, UK. She is currently working on the DACHA study (developing research resources and minimum data set for care homes' adoption and use), funded by the National Institute for Health Research, which addresses the need to develop robust systems for the benefit of care home residents. Previously, she worked as a teaching fellow in the Department of Digital Humanities at King's College London, UK. Gizdem completed her PhD at the London School of Economics, under the Information Systems and Innovation Faculty Research Group. Her research interests include health information systems, health services research, ageing studies, policy research, and qualitative methods.

Routledge Advances in Health and Social Policy

Planning Later Life
Bioethics and Public Health in Ageing Societies
Edited by Mark Schweda, Larissa Pfaller, Kai Brauer, Frank Adloff and Silke Schicktanz

Effective Interventions for Unemployed Young People in Europe
Social Innovation or Paradigm Shift?
Edited by Tomas Sirovatka and Henk Spies

Social Research in Health and Illness
Case-Based Approaches
Constantinos N. Phellas and Costas S. Constantinou

Ethnic Identity and US Immigration Policy Reform
American Citizenship and Belonging amongst Hispanic Immigrants
Maria del Mar Farina

Research and Evaluation in Community, Health and Social Care Settings
Experiences from Practice
Edited by Suzanne Guerin, Nóirín Hayes and Sinead McNally

Critical Discourses of Old Age and Telecare Technologies
Gizdem Akdur

For more information about this series, please visit: www.routledge.com/Routledge-Advances-in-Health-and-Social-Policy/book-series/RAHSP

Critical Discourses of Old Age and Telecare Technologies

Gizdem Akdur

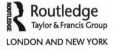
LONDON AND NEW YORK

First published 2020
by Routledge
2 Park Square, Milton Park, Abingdon, Oxon OX14 4RN

and by Routledge
52 Vanderbilt Avenue, New York, NY 10017

Routledge is an imprint of the Taylor & Francis Group, an informa business

© 2020 Gizdem Akdur

The right of Gizdem Akdur to be identified as author of this work has been asserted by her in accordance with sections 77 and 78 of the Copyright, Designs and Patents Act 1988.

All rights reserved. No part of this book may be reprinted or reproduced or utilised in any form or by any electronic, mechanical, or other means, now known or hereafter invented, including photocopying and recording, or in any information storage or retrieval system, without permission in writing from the publishers.

Trademark notice: Product or corporate names may be trademarks or registered trademarks, and are used only for identification and explanation without intent to infringe.

British Library Cataloguing-in-Publication Data
A catalogue record for this book is available from the British Library

Library of Congress Cataloging-in-Publication Data
A catalog record has been requested for this book

ISBN: 978-0-367-46512-4 (hbk)
ISBN: 978-1-003-02921-2 (ebk)

Typeset in Times New Roman
by codeMantra

Contents

List of figures	vi
List of tables	vii
Acknowledgements	viii
1 Introduction: connecting old age with telecare	1
2 A general review of old age and telecare	5
3 A critical enquiry into discourses and the identity of old age	58
4 Conclusions and future directions	112
References	116
Appendices	129
Index	146

Figures

2.1	Grand discourses of old age	18
2.2	How telecare works	20
3.1	Responses to the question "Services that could be made available – which are relevant to you and which would you use?" from people with and without longer-term conditions	70
3.2	A subjectivity formation model created by merging modes of objectification with Hacking's looping effects	74
3.3	Dividing the aspects of primary themes into further overarching themes	89
3.4	Classifying discourses, processes, and relations under the grand discourses of old age	102
3.5	Overlapping discourses, processes, and relations between the grand discourses of old age	103

Tables

2.1	List of key concepts and constructs	55
3.1	List of themes: forewords	86
3.2	List of themes: visual representations	87
3.3	List of identified discourses and processes relating to old age	101

Acknowledgements

This book is based on my doctoral thesis, submitted to the London School of Economics in January 2019. I would like to dedicate it to my grandparents, Dervise and Halil.

1 Introduction
Connecting old age with telecare

Old age has a history of problematisations in Britain, through which certain narratives of old age have been produced and sustained. In the early 1900s, ageing was "discovered" as a social issue, and "old age" was created as a separate group (Phillipson, 1998). Until the 1920s, older people formed an emerging group that was differentiated based on their poverty as well as their status in relation to work. Starting in the 1940s, the vocabulary around ageing expanded because the welfare state established post-WWII, from 1945 onwards, started offering pensions for those of retirement age, as well as offering healthcare services for older people in a distinct way via the newly founded National Health Service (NHS) (founded in 1948). With medical and technological advancements extending life spans over the century, by the 1970s, an optimistic view of retirement was created that considered it as a major stage in life; depictions of this age group as endowed with leisure time, energy, and spare funds for activities and luxuries led to the emergent conceptualisation of a new kind of target demographic: the "gold in grey" consumers (Minkler, 1991).

These coincided with Thatcher-era policies, in the 1980s, which encouraged increased privatisation (e.g. of homes and various services), cuts to government spending on social care, and the dismantling of strong unions, of which NHS staff had been a large part. In the 1980s, public interest in ageing issues was growing alongside anxieties about the funding crisis of the welfare state (Gilleard and Higgs, 2014). Old age was seen as an economic burden, with the dichotomising vision of struggling young working people funding older dependents developing. In the 1990s, the status of older people faced destabilisation due to uncertainty about the provision of pensions. Old age was increasingly interpreted via financial justifications in an era of demographic constraints and increased outsourcing to private sector providers. Today, old age faces similar interpretations, which are carried forward by the dominant historical discourses.

The making of the aged body and the older population into the central focus of scientific knowledge and political practices has its origins in the period during which age became a regulatory theme in family, schooling, work, and retirement. The existing discourses of old age are thus products of the ways in which bodies and populations have been historically problematised through the regulation of age. Three grand narratives of old age have been identified by critical gerontology and old age studies, which are still relevant in the postmodern life course. These are: (1) the biomedical model that perceives ageing as a pathological problem and ties ageing to those discourses of decline, abnormality, deterioration, and dependency; (2) the consumer culture that perceives older people as a new group of homogeneous, financially secure, and powerful consumers; and (3) managerialism in social work that perceives older people in terms of risk (Featherstone and Hepworth, 1989; Phillipson, 1998; Phillipson and Biggs, 1998; Biggs and Powell, 2001; Powell and Biggs, 2004).

This book combines two distinct subjects of research: (1) old age and (2) telecare technologies, which are known as the remote care services for older people. Due to the challenges presented by ageing populations and the consequentially increasing demand for health and social care services, technological care has seen a global rise in recent decades. In the UK, the scope of telecare services has been growing since the 1990s through the increasing number of government policies and strategies created about these technologies. In the past decade, the UK Government has been advocating the widespread adoption of telecare services, and the technology industry has been presenting new technological innovations to enhance well-being and health as the population ages. Large state-sponsored trials of telecare were conducted in the early 2010s, from which ambiguous results were published in medicine studies about the effectiveness of telecare (Cartwright et al., 2013; Henderson et al., 2013, 2014; Hirani et al., 2013; Steventon et al., 2012, 2013). Nevertheless, the pervasiveness of telecare services has been consistently growing, and more local authorities have been offering these services to their residents. Telecare information systems occupy a greater part of public social care policies, and thus they create a new domain in which old age narratives can find their place. Older people are the primary users and stakeholders of telecare technologies, and are processed, interpreted, classified, and organised within these information systems.

There has been a cohort of research about care technologies from different fields, such as information systems, health services research, medicine, and sociology. The sociological studies of old age and care technologies have been mainly influenced by Michel Foucault's school of thought, and they reflect on such topics as governmentality, control, surveillance, and ethics (Powell and Biggs, 2004; Schermer, 2009; Guta et al., 2012; Sorell and Draper, 2012). Foucauldian theories and frameworks have been influential in the domain of old age studies; power and discourse analysis has been the focus in this area of research. This is because discourses concerning old age are available in the structures and institutions found in everyday life, including the policies and politics of the governments. With regard to this, there are certain narratives of old age that can arise out of policies that concern telecare. These texts and practices reveal "explicit and implicit ways of positioning older people" (NCPOP, 2009, p. 4), meaning that older people are given particular identities.

Outline

In this book, I will systematically demonstrate how an old age identity is constructed based on discourses emerging from telecare-related national policies and how these discourses are closely linked with the historically existing grand discourses of old age. I will explore those enactments or alterations of the grand discourses of old age in relation to telecare, and explain the effects that discourses of old age have on the old age identity. The question, *'How is the identity of old age constituted in relation to telecare technologies?'*, is essential to guiding the critical enquiry undertaken in this book.

Chapter 2 reviews the literature of gerontology and old age studies, and it creates an association between old age and telecare. Telecare is placed in the field of information systems and other fields, and theoretical insights are revealed with regard to how these technologies can be linked to the problematisations of old age. A set of concepts and constructs are also defined in Chapter 2. Telecare information systems are recognised as complex systems that consist of technological, political, social, and economic components. Finally, the chapter also introduces analytical tools and contextualises Foucault's *modes of objectification* and discourse analysis to guide the critical enquiry of government policies in the next chapter.

Chapter 3 presents the history of the NHS and telecare policies to contextualise the state of social care services in England. It answers the question outlined earlier by applying the *modes of objectification* to the policies. The chapter presents the discourses of old age and structural relations that are mediated through policies related to old age and telecare. Then, these are placed within the *grand discourses* of old age to reflect on how the grand discourses have been sustained and expanded. At the end, old age identity is defined by reflecting on the discourses and processes that are historically sustained, emerging, disrupted, or dissolving.

Chapter 4 presents an overview and concluding remarks whilst discussing how contributions can be made to policy. Finally, possibilities for future research are outlined.

2 A general review of old age and telecare

This chapter starts with the introduction of the premises upon which the problematisations of old age were built, and which narratives of old age are produced and sustained. Then, I reflect upon telecare technologies, their relation to older people, and different approaches used in telecare research. And finally, I introduce my analytical 'toolbox', which will make the analysis of government policies possible.

Ageing and old age

A brief history of old age in Britain

The idea of old people as a separate group and the creation of the old age pension are the products of the late 1800s. In Britain, state pensions began in 1870s, and non-contributory pension legislation came into effect in 1908. Prior to this period, provision for older people was not differentiated from provision for people with sicknesses (Slater, 1930). The political environment at this point considered old age as a problem that required new social policies. In the early 1900s, ageing was 'discovered' as a social issue. Until the 1920s, older people formed an emerging group that was differentiated based on their poverty as well as their status in relation to work. Poverty and marginalisation were common occurrences in the lives of older people, which led to the construction of a framework of older age that was based on similar occurrences and experiences. Consequently, old age was constructed around "harsh or softer versions of dependency" (Phillipson, 1998), such as the concept of older people as a problem population, or of older people as deserving of a reward for their past contributions to society.

In Britain, several social rights were gained with the start of the post-war (after WWII) period welfare state, with a growing idea of social inclusion. Starting in the 1940s, the vocabulary around ageing expanded, because the welfare state was offering pensions and health services in a distinct way compared to the previous periods, when old age had been constructed around poverty and dependency. Until the 1950s, old age was a social status of white heterosexual able-bodied men. In the institutionalised life course of this society, the modernist model of social structure provided the boundaries of the labour force – and chronological age, rather than corporeal age, was taken as the legitimised means through which men could exit this labour force. The state was the main provider of support when this chronological limit was reached, enabling men to be freed from labour. Therefore, men's lives were more or less divided into two frames of status: (1) one of 'working age' and (2) the other 'old age', which was inevitably framed by the former (Phillipson, 1998). This strict marking of men's lives by their chronological age did not follow the same fashion for the women's life course. A woman's life was defined by individual circumstances, her health status, and personal relationships (marriage, motherhood, widowhood, etc.) rather than by the economic system, as was the case for men (Gilleard and Higgs, 2014).

In the post-war welfare state period, the modern government was given the central responsibility over older people for the first time, and it did so in a novel way through developing a moral framework. The identity of older people was influenced by this framework, and it evolved in various ways with emerging ideas such as 'active retirement'. Retirement as a positive experience took time to spread beyond a certain class and group of retirees. At the beginning of the post-war period, retirement was seen as a psychosocial crisis, with increased morbidity and mortality rates (Phillipson, 1993). These could have been the consequence of loss of work-based relationships and loss of self-esteem with age. However, by the 1970s a more positive view of retirement was created. The understanding of retirement as a major stage in life with active lifestyles was fostered in this period.

In the 1960s, after the high point and subsequent dissolution of the 'first modernity' were experienced, a new 'normativity of diversity' (Beck, 2007; Gilleard and Higgs, 2014) started to replace the former cultural arrangements. The body started having other possible identities, and new embodiment types – new forms of social agency – were realised upon the features of the corporeal. This made possible alternative lifestyles as distinct from the standardised lifestyles of the first modernity. With respect to the identity of older people, the society now found itself in a period of crisis. Between the 1950s and the early 1970s, the institutions of the welfare state and retirement were the main enabling forces that were considered to secure old age. By the 1980s, however, the development of earlier retirement plans caused the state financial distress. This situation was exacerbated by the stagnating growth of the welfare state in the mid-1970s. Contributing factors such as a rise in inflation and unemployment as well as a slow economic growth challenged the principles of spending on the welfare state. Following this, the older people's welfare state started to erode in the late 1980s. The expansionist welfare reforms of the 1960s and 1970s shifted towards plans to privatise the provision of pensions, and to separate the better off from the poorest by targeting the resources on the poor.

The nature of discussions revolving around old age in the Britain of the 1980s was influenced by such factors as growing public interest in ageing issues, the crisis of funding for the welfare state, and concerns regarding its future. These factors made old age enter an arena of ambivalent points of debate: on the one hand, growing old signified liberation; on the other, older people were seen as a marginalised group of the population (Phillipson, 1998). The problems with public spending were more openly constructed around old age as an economic burden, and the restraints in social services and healthcare expenditures were increasingly justified through this. By the 1990s, several crises were observed that were related to the status of older people in this society, arising from doubts surrounding the system of retirement and from views challenging the assumptions about the welfare state. These changes started to gradually result in ideologies that defined older people as a burden to society (Phillipson, 1998).

The welfare state and old age

The nature of demographic change has always been a concern for Western societies, and it has been problematised with costs and burdens that these changes would bring. Increasing expenses of healthcare services, and the ageing population becoming an unwelcome burden on society were the kind of doubts that arose with demographic changes in society. In the United Kingdom, a succession of social policy changes took place after the Second World War: (1) this started with a welfare system, (2) turned to marketisation in the Thatcher era, and (3) shifted towards European notions of social inclusion in the late 1990s (Phillipson and Biggs, 1998; Biggs and Powell, 2001). Each change has had implications on the public discourses that construct ageing.

In the 1950s, the goal of achieving security in old age was something that the population worked towards through the means of maintaining full employment and creating channels for secure retirement. However, these ideals were falling apart by the 1990s, with the removal of full employment goals and the deindexation[1] of pensions from wages that caused a loss in value. These factors were also supplemented with the increasing number of workers who were disinclined or reluctant to pay tax increases to support benefits for vulnerable groups such as older people, and in so doing were breaking the 'intergenerational contract'[2] (Phillipson, 1998) of the pensions system.

Starting in the 1950s, the construction of an identity in retirement developed within society at large, and this was studied in the research literature. The new patterns of consumption developed by retired people in areas such as leisure and education were slowly becoming subjects of study in the 1980s. Middle age was continuously redefined to be a more youthful phase in life, during which time individuals are managing their consumption and life-style opportunities in order "to enable their retirement to be a progressive set of options and choices – a phase in which the individual is presented as still moving within the social space, still learning, [and] investing in cultural capital" (Featherstone, 1987, p. 134). The services sector also started recognising the significance of the market for 50-plus-year-old individuals. The development of private sheltered housings, retirement magazines, and specialised holiday companies are a few examples of this recognition.

This changing vision of retirement was contributing towards the reconstruction of the identity of an older person. Whereas in the 1950s, retirement was seen as an impairment to mental health, from the 1980s onwards, it was increasingly considered to be a pathway to fulfilment, where people achieve those lifestyles that were not possible within the workplace (Phillipson, 1998). These views existed from the late 1960s until the 1980s. When concerns of the 1990s surrounding high unemployment rates and dependent populations started to arise, tensions developed in the social relationships between retired older people and the rest of the society. During the 1980s and 1990s, the expansion of a 'medical gaze'[3] could also be observed in policy debates concerned with shrinking public budgets and fears surrounding the dissolution of an intergenerational social contract, which was considered to be the foundation of the post-war welfare state (Phillipson, 1998; Biggs and Powell, 2001).

Even though during the Thatcher and post-Thatcher years, the welfare state expenditures had grown, the scope of this spending in relation to the old population was reduced. Between the mid-1970s and

1990s there were reductions in the amount of care facilities for older people, in bed capacities of hospitals, and in the number of acute beds, almost half of which were accounted for by older people (Phillipson, 1998). It has been documented that the privatisation of services once undertaken by the government, increasing class divisions in access to services, and service fragmentation were factors contributing to the crisis in community care in the late twentieth century. Estes and Linkins (1997) refer to the separation between government and the services that the government funds with the term 'hollow state'. The hollow state typically contracts outs its provision to the private sector and keeps for itself the monitoring and inspection responsibilities. In the UK, there has been an increase in the overall private spending, and an increasing practice of hollow state since the 1980s.

Both the institutions of the welfare state and of retirement contributed to the social construction of an emerging identity of old age. The welfare state itself offered a set of values for being an older person. But, with the removal of the foundations of retirement and welfare state, the meaning of old age was becoming obscure and less secure. This sort of change in the history of old age has had effects on the lives of older people. Social gerontology and the sociology of ageing have grown substantially since the 1980s to study experiences and relationships in older people's lives. Prior to this, most accounts of ageing defined it as a universal, non-reversible, and deleterious process of decline (Strehler, 1962). Gerontology has engaged with ageing in a way in which ageing has been either reified as a marker of individual achievement, or inserted within a social care or biomedical narrative wherein health or disability statuses are key criteria of judgement (Gilleard and Higgs, 2014).

The uncertainty about the provision of pensions, as a result of the dissolving institution of retirement, is one of the key elements in the destabilisation of old age (Phillipson, 1998). The unravelling of retirement has historically also been focussed on unravelling the financial arrangements associated with welfare state. These changes and reforms in the arrangements of the welfare state and social security have increasingly linked growing old to insecurities in later life. Emerging institutions of late modernity play a role in reshaping conceptions of growing old, in which 'alarmist views' of demographic change and ideological pressure upon older people were developed (Phillipson, 1998).

The frameworks that older people previously relied on for support were transforming; whereas the idea of the welfare state between the 1950s and 1970s embodied a sense of 'moral progress' with the centrality of older people (Leonard, 1997), the status of old age shifted in later decades. From the 1990s onwards, the vision of old age was interpreted via its financial justifications in an era of demographic constraints, causing conflict between generations and anxieties about the equitability of the welfare state.

Modernity, postmodernity, and old age

With the advent of modernity, the hospital became a specialised supporting structure for the medicalisation of older people as 'patients' (Katz, 1996). The medicalisation of hospitals and the production of medical knowledge were the products of the rise of Western rationality, the logic that leads social and economic relationships in Western societies to be arranged based on context and the debates surrounding old age. Distinct modern categories, such as notions of the 'sick' and 'ill patient', arose out of classifications of this rationality (Katz, 1996; Powell and Biggs, 2004).

What is defined by Giddens (1991) as 'late modernity' is a move towards a postmodern society, in which traditional institutions and routines are abandoned. In postmodernity, people are responsible for negotiating their lifestyles and making their own choices about how they want to conduct their lives; mechanisms of self-identity both shape and are shaped by the institutions of modernity, where the self becomes a reflexive project with continuously revised narratives (Giddens, 1991). These mechanisms operate on flexibilities and choices by replacing the rigidity of traditional styles. Based on Beck's (1992) conceptualisation, social change comprises three stages: (a) pre-modernity, (b) simple (first) modernity, and (c) reflexive (second) modernity/postmodernity.[4]

Reflexive/second modernity or postmodernity (c) offers the key component of individualisation as its foundation of social change. It is individualisation that largely breaks down traditional structures, such as church and village communities that existed in pre-modernity (Lash, 1994). In simple or first modernity (b), these archaic structures give way to trade unions, welfare state, class as a structure etc. by being partly influenced by the individualisation process. Two important developments can be noted for the period that coincides with the dissolution of the first (simple) modernity and gives momentum to the society to take a *somatic turn* (Gilleard and Higgs, 2014). (1) One is the significance that the society started placing on the 'embodiment of identities', and (2) the next is the extension of 'embodied practices' that served to realise these embodied identities. These practices refer to the practices of self-care and self-expression mediated by society.

Further individualisation sets agency free from these social structures of simple modernity (Lash, 1994). This means that reflexive modernity separates individuals from collective structures. Ecological concerns, the crisis of the nuclear family, and the changes in the class structures of today are the results of this individualisation. Even though the dissolution of boundaries in postmodernism (referred to as 'late modernity' by some authors) leads to a recognition of multiplicities in social life, it has been argued that postmodern thought makes the view in relation to ageing narrower because it primarily focusses on flexibilities and choices while dismissing the inequalities associated with class, gender, ethnic background, etc. – the elements that continue to shape older people's lives (Phillipson, 1998).

These developments raise issues for those institutions around which old age was constructed. For example, retirement policies were formed around "a society based on mass production and mass institutions" (Phillipson, 1998, p. 46). As the changes to modernity create distinct types of ageing – with respect to social relationships after the termination of work – distinct types of identities in older age are produced. In what has been described as the 'modernisation of ageing' by Featherstone and Hepworth (1989) there are three key characteristics that make ageing different in the late modernity/postmodern period: (1) the frequent occurrence of youthful images of retirement; (2) the social construction of middle age (creating a part of life known as 'mid-life'); and (3) a period of extended mid-life that includes states of complex transitional states, personal growth, and development.

Although these changes in the modernity of ageing generate positive images of ageing and older people, it is debatable whether these areas can be transgressed and afforded only by people with wealth (Featherstone and Hepworth, 1989). Despite the production of affirmative social images of old age, it is argued that most older people might face the negative sides of ageing due to the disorganised and relatively insecure institutions, such as retirement, that are being broken down with the structures of late modernity (Phillipson, 1998). Such debates concerning relationships between structures and old age created in literature somewhat pessimistic views of the ways in which old age has been classified through decades. Phillipson has stated that

> the label of 'older person' has diminished rather than enhanced the lives of those to whom it is applied (...) with the welfare state actually contributing rather less to the status of older people than its founders might reasonably have hoped.
> (Phillipson, 1998, p. 123)

The language that focussed on old age in the post-war and late modernity periods contributed to generating an oppressive vision of ageing, by turning older people into a marginal group. By taking into account the positive consumerist views of old age, Moody suggests that

> the rise of the nursing homes industry does not empower older people to make decisions about their lives. Instead, the elderly become a new class of consumer subject to the expanding domination by professionals in [what Estes has termed] the 'Ageing Enterprise'. Instead of freedom, we have the 'colonization' of the life world in old age, and the last stage is emptied of any meaning beyond sheer biological survival.
>
> (Moody, 1992, p. 115)

These views have been widely studied in critical gerontology, the field that critically approaches old age studies and traditional gerontology.

The examination of knowledge about the *body* as a site of power relations coincides with the rise of issues related to identities in the second half of the twentieth century. As the body became distinctly embodied in the late modernity, it became an arena for self-care and for practices of self-transformation (Foucault, 1994a). What Foucault termed the 'clinical gaze' constituted the foundation of new forms of power/knowledge relations by which normal/abnormal, illness/health were defined. New forms of power by the medical sciences arise when individuals are both subjects and objects of their own knowledge (Foucault, 1975). A Foucauldian perspective on the study of ageing can be captured by replacing the word 'sex/sexuality' with 'age' in his phrases on sexuality: "[Age] appeared as an extremely unstable pathological field: a surface of repercussion for other ailments, but also the focus of a specific nosography,[5] that of instincts, tendencies, images, pleasure and conduct" (Foucault, 1980a, p. 67; Katz, 1996, p. 7). Katz uses another statement from *The History of Sexuality* (Foucault, 1980a), to indicate similarities between old age and sexuality:

> [Age] is not the most intractable element in power relations, but rather one of those endowed with the greatest instrumentality: useful for the greatest number of manoeuvres and capable of serving as a point of support, as a linchpin, for the most varied strategies.
>
> (p. 103; Katz, 1996, p. 7)

The individualisation process that has occurred as part of late modernity is echoed in the shift away from the public provision of services.

This inextricably affects the identity of older people, because growing old as a collective experience is transformed into an individual one in this process. Here, emphasis on ageing individuals rather than on the social responsibilities of an ageing society becomes primary; the understanding of the crisis of ageing is associated with "how individuals rather than societies handle the demands associated with social ageing" (Phillipson, 1998, p. 119). The institutional spaces occupied by older individuals have transformed as a result of developments in late modernity, which include the identities defined through institutions of welfare, retirement, and family. With the wave of economic anxieties and concerns about the welfare state in the 1990s, the view of old age involved a particular emphasis on dependence on these institutions. It was clear that the re-definitions of old age during the post-war welfare period could not escape the view of old people as a burden, as seen in the use of labels such as 'the elderly infirm', 'the aged', and 'the frail ambulant' (Cottam, 1954, p. 7). This view has carried on into subsequent decades, in the form of institutional ageism, and it has contributed to turning older people into a specifically classified group again and again.

Starting in the 2000s, a theoretical current named 'Foucauldian gerontology' has risen. Its aim has been to understand "how ageing is socially constructed by discourses used by professions and disciplines in order to control and regulate the experiences of older people and to legitimise powerful narratives afforded to age by such groups" (Powell and Biggs, 2003). The use of Foucault's narrative in gerontology offered a novel way to problematise knowledge systems and break the assumptions taken for granted about ageing. Even though there have only been a handful of studies utilising such methods, the aspect of 'historical investigation' has gradually enabled more scholars to use history as a way to diagnose current social conditions.

Problematisation of old age

Problematisation, as described in a Foucauldian approach, "signifies the disciplinary practices that transform a realm of human existence into a crisis of thought" (Katz, 1996, p. 9). The problematisations in the gerontological field can be characterised to be of individual adjustment and of population ageing. In critical gerontology, Foucauldian approaches are used to study the medicalisation of the body wherein the aged body is transformed into a pathological subject, and the governmentality of the population, which looks at the discursive technologies that differentiate the aged population as a special kind. This kind is mainly characterised in political discourses by their neediness (Katz, 1996). Additionally, Foucault's lens creates a shift in gerontology by repositioning the focus from how the history and the knowledge of gerontology has problematised old age to how the subjectification of old age has enabled the formation of this knowledge possible.

From Foucault's perspective, the study of the formation of gerontological knowledge within specific power/knowledge practices and subjectivities surpasses traditional histories of progress in official knowledge production. This view asserts that the apparatuses used in gerontological human sciences – such as surveys, theories, texts, codes, and models – are disciplinary techniques that compose the knowledge and the subjects of old age. The making of the aged body and the older population into the central focus of scientific knowledge and political practices has its origins in the period when age became a regulatory theme in family, schooling, work, and retirement. Existing discourses of old age are, therefore, products of the ways in which bodies and populations have been historically problematised through the regulation of age.

The postmodern life course, as depicted in the work of Featherstone and Hepworth (1989), blurred the traditional boundaries of chronology of life and integrated the periods of life that were segregated previously. This postmodern shift from universalism to fragmentation created the 'consumer culture' (Featherstone and Wernick, 1995; Powell and Biggs, 2004). Medical indices of decline were slowly substituted with the agelessness of the 'consumers' wherein age was no longer a chronological marker. As a new group of consumers – or "gold in grey" (Minkler, 1991) – older people are characterised as a homogeneous, financially secure, powerful interest group. However, this discourse coexists with another grand narrative: the older population is seen to be the dependent burden on healthcare programs and welfare, and a drain on society's resources.

The biomedical model that perceives ageing as a pathological problem ties ageing to those discourses of decline, abnormality, deterioration, and dependency (Phillipson, 1998; Powell and Biggs, 2003). These master narratives of consumer agelessness, and biological decline and dependency may seem to promote contradictory narratives, yet they are interrelated. "They are contradictory in their relation to notions of autonomy, independence, and dependency on others, yet linked through the importance of techniques for maintenance (…) via medicalized bodily control" (Biggs and Powell, 2001, p. 95). Biggs (2001) argues that a shift in policy interest is occurring in the UK that replaces the narrative of decline in old age with one that promotes active and successful ageing and anti-ageism. Anti-dependency is becoming a characteristic in these policies. This change is "an attempt to shape acceptable forms of ageing whilst encouraging older people to self-monitor their own success at conforming to the new paradigm" (Powell and Biggs, 2003) through the adoption of technologies that enable self-modification and self-scrutiny. This means that the rhetoric of burden and dependency in later life finds its way in the new rhetoric of anti-dependency.

Biggs and Powell (2001) argue that the focus on medicalised bodily control and adoption of consumer lifestyles has obscured a third grand discourse on ageing, which has been strong in Europe and the UK: the discourse that associates old age with social welfare. From the nineteenth century onwards, transformations that took place concerning social welfare were associated with moral panics about the family (Jones, 1983). Professionalisation of social work developed in the nexus of public and private spaces and was seen as a benevolent solution to a major problem, namely: how can the state ensure the health of family members who are dependent by promoting it as natural to care for them in the family sphere, without direct intervention into families (Hirst, 1981)? This solution situated social work between the state and the individual families. While medicine drew heavily on technical knowledge, social work started drawing from the fields of psychoanalysis and the social sciences. Social work became a vehicle through which the attributes and qualities of individuals could be managed and improved. Its legitimacy was dependent upon its relationship with the welfare state, and soon social work became prominent in the development of social regulation techniques – which can be characterised as forms of surveillance, discipline, and normalisation (Foucault, 1977; Biggs and Powell, 2001).

Even though the size of the dependent population was forecasted to remain the same over five decades from the 1970s to the 2020s (Patel, 1990; Biggs and Powell, 2001), the change in the future dependent population's composition (less children and more older people) was the source of the panic. With older people as the centre of social work's agenda, social work narratives started paralleling the medicalised rhetoric of burdensome decline in old age. Intervention by professionals was increasingly allowed when the conduct of an older person was believed to be a hazard to themselves or to those around them, and the caring profession drew from psychoanalytical discourses that pathologised older age. It constructed an image of older people as 'demanding' and 'always complaining' (Irvine, 1954), and thus the narrative of old age as burden and attached notions of dependency were reinforced through social workers who were the gatekeepers to the provision of social care (Biggs and Powell, 2001). This narrative of dependency was also increasingly articulated in state policies. Biggs and Powell argue that the arrival of managerialism in the United Kingdom in the 1990s marked a shift in social welfare towards control and surveillance (Biggs and Powell, 2001; Powell and Biggs, 2000). They depict it as a result of the shift from the welfare state, which created top-down social policies to manage dependent populations, to the *post-welfare* and *neoliberal* state, in which social regulations depend on bottom-up structures. Powell and Biggs reflect on this change: "central control has been replaced by local power; management systems are inspired by consumer and market models; there is a reliance on risk assessment; and an increase in the discourses of a 'politics of participation' and 'social inclusion'" (2000, p. 4). The management of old age through the consolidation of managerial power gave special attention to reforms in welfare apparatuses. In the UK, these reforms were backed up by alarmist arguments based on demographics, which were imposed by the central government (Warnes, 1996; Powell and Biggs, 2000). Care managerialism was a move away from direct care towards assessment and monitoring on the basis of 'the old age problem'.

The aim of such reforms is to reduce the financial burden of age on the state and on the family through economic privatisation and through turning older people into active consumers, whose empowerment through 'choice' (of services) is marked as an end. It has been stated that scientific dominance, supplemented with financial narratives, has been gradually growing in relation to the provision of care; a powerful and pervasive discourse of 'old people as consumers' has been formed through the models of care management (Powell and Biggs, 2000). At the local level in the UK, the shift to a managerial model in social services has been influential in challenging the dependency of the older population by promoting empowerment through choice, and through initiating new relationships, such as the partnerships between professional service providers and older people.

The mixed economy of welfare that was introduced through increasing managerialism in care highlights the incorporation of market forces into the planning and provision of services. It embodies a multitude of political agendas in a bid to control financial resources, improve services, change how local authorities work, establish new techniques for resource allocations, and reduce public provision of services, etc. Their idealised concepts of *choice* and *empowerment* for older people have been contested because the associated changes are argued to have widened the sphere of collective control and regulation (Powell and Biggs, 2000). In the same vein, the transformation of older people into consumers can lead collective concerns to be given a backseat in favour of individual transactions. That is because such narratives of empowerment can transform into politically neutral and individual questions of *satisfaction* with products and services, rather than an encapsulation of collective accounts (Estes and Linkins, 1997; Biggs and Powell, 2001).

This means that managerial power can have an impact on old age identities through the care policies of the state and the practices of social service institutions. Because managerialism primarily relies on risk assessments, this model results in the intensification of the inspecting gaze. Foucault argues that when individuals are taken as 'cases', they are "described, judged, measured, compared with others" so that they can "be trained or corrected, classified, normalised, excluded" (1977, p. 191). 'Assessment' as a disciplinary technique aims to describe, judge, measure, and compare older people with the use of norms and by "imposing new delimitations on them" (Foucault, 1977, p. 184). This type of standardisation creates an individualising effect that promotes homogeneity in the identity of old age (Powell and Biggs, 2000) by "making it possible to measure gaps, to determine levels, to fix specialities and to render the differences useful by fitting them to one another" (Foucault, 1977, p. 185).

Summary

I have reviewed the construction of old age through the knowledge production of sciences and the state. The grand discourses that problematise old age are given particular emphasis. These narratives can be summarised as follows.

These grand narratives form the basis of the analysis to be undertaken in this book. My aim is to: (1) explore the enactments or alterations of the grand discourses of old age within the domain of telecare information systems (IS) and (2) examine the effects that the grand discourses and other discourses of old age have on the identity of old age. The next section will review research conducted on social care and telecare technologies, because telecare technologies in the UK mainly target the ageing population, and the studies of telecare explicitly or implicitly address the concerns of old age.

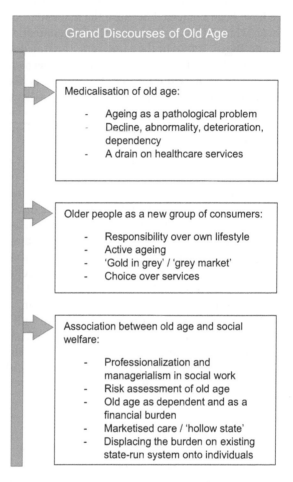

Figure 2.1 Grand discourses of old age (own illustration, 2018).

Telecare technologies in the United Kingdom

In the late 1990s, the UK government directed their initiatives towards developing wired communities in order to promote health and independence, modernising care services, and delivering value for money (Department of Health, 1998). With this idea, telecare services emerged in a network of information systems. While enabling older people to live safely and independently in their homes, telecare strategies were expected to be aligned with a wide range of healthcare, social care, and housing-related government initiatives. After the recognition of telecare technologies in an information strategy white paper (NHS Executive – DOH, 1998), the government invested in extending the use of telecare technologies at a national level with the introduction of various initiatives.

In the UK, telecare has always been defined in relation to *community alarms*. Alarm systems have been available in the UK for over 50 years and were originally designed for the use of older people (Miskelly, 2001). The first and second generation of community alarms have been designed for the purposes of risk management and security provision (Sixsmith and Sixsmith, 2008). First generation community alarm services were initially launched in sheltered housing to ensure the safety of people when wardens were off the premises. Community alarms were designed to offer a simple model of raising an alarm in a call centre or to alert the wardens with the push of a button or the pulling of a cord. Community alarm services widely spread over the country over the next decades; soon they were used as portable alarm units in individual homes. These systems evolved into second-generation systems in order to respond to problems that could not be recognised before. Identifying abnormal or unusual patterns in the everyday lives of older people became the motive behind this evolution that led to telecare. Telecare systems are comprised of: (a) a 24-hour telecommunications link to control centres, (b) records systems to monitor alerts and to log new data, (c) environmental sensors (smoke, temperature, gas, etc.), (d) passive sensors (bed pressure sensors, door opening sensors, etc.), and (e) intelligent home unit devices to link the sensors together (Sixsmith and Sixsmith, 2008). These features of telecare have differentiated telecare services from the first-generation alarm services. They also have enabled higher volumes of data collection from the service users due to the increasing number of links with more devices and sensors. Even though community alarms and telecare services coexist today, there has been a gradual shift towards telecare systems.

The logical shift for community alarm services in the UK has been towards more proactive forms of telecare. This includes passive alarms and sensors that offer a monitoring service and alerts the call centre automatically without the need to press a button when hazards arise (Curry et al., 2002). Improvements in monitoring systems and advancements in the development of various smart sensors and intelligent home units have been the main changes to the community alarm services over the past decade. Additionally, the subject of falls prevention has become an increasingly important area of research in the UK. As a major cause of injury in old age, falls are an expense to

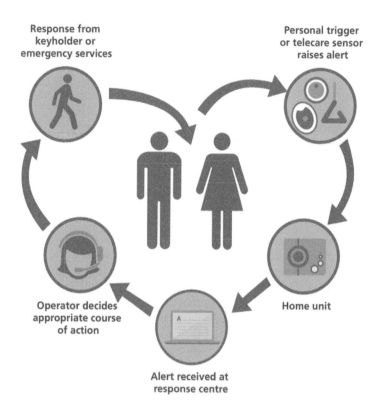

Figure 2.2 How telecare works. The image is from NHS England's 'NHS Long Term Conditions Flyer' (2012, p. 2). Licensed under the Open Government Licence for Public Sector Information v3.0 – http://www.nationalarchives.gov.uk/doc/open-government-licence/version/3/.

the healthcare system, an estimated £2.3 billion per year. Based on a National Institute for Health and Care Excellence report, people aged 65 and older have the highest risk of falling; 30% of people older than 65, and half of people older than 80 fall at least once a year in England (NICE, 2013). The phenomenon of falling at an older age is also argued to be an indicator of larger issues that involve social support, independent living, health policy, and housing, and is often a threshold that marks the life between independent housing and hospitalisation (Katz, 2010). Preventive and monitoring-based solutions have therefore gained momentum, in line with increasing anxieties over independence and assistance and with advancements in technologies.

Telecare refers to living independently in one's own home with the application and help of ICTs. As well as assisting in the delivery of services, telecare maintains the security and safety of older people in their houses. As Loader et al. (2008) notes, there is a distinction between the two types of telecare systems: (1) one is designed for assessment and information sharing, and (2) the other is designed for risk management. However, the terminology that the Department of Health uses in their report (Department of Health, 2009) shows that the above distinctions are grouped under two separate titles: risk management services as *telecare*; information sharing and assessment services as *telehealth*. This is how both services are described (Department of Health, 2009): the Telehealth systems allow individuals with chronic conditions such as obstructive pulmonary disease (COPD), diabetes, heart failure or a mixture of these conditions to exchange data (e.g. blood levels) with healthcare professionals using a set of products such as blood pressure monitors, glucometers, and weighing scales. On the other hand, telecare systems focus on people who are in constant need of health and social care services for support, and are "facing difficulties carrying their current burden of responsibilities" (Department of Health, 2009). Telecare technologies are a combination of wireless sensors and alarms that track the changes in an individual's activities and raise a call in the event of emergencies, such as a fire or a fall. Personal alarms, temperature sensors, gas/water detectors, and bed occupancy sensors are only a few examples of the products that are used as a part of telecare services. The most important distinguishing factor between the two services is the matter of information systems (IS): the centralised and continuously monitored systems of telecare consist of more refined forms of information storage, retrieval, and filtering, and link to several actors responsible for care at once.

Telecare initiatives in search of more cost-effective ways of caring for older people and people with complex long-term conditions (Sanders et al., 2012) have become a bigger part of the Department of Health's agenda in recent years. These services are more relied upon to bring major implications for health and social care services by transforming the order of care and extending the reach of healthcare outside of consulting rooms and hospitals (Oudshoorn, 2011). There have been various pilot projects at local councils across the country – including notable projects in London, Surrey, Durham, and a few others – that were conducted by the social services of the related councils. In 2004, the Government introduced the Preventative Technology Grant whose aim was to initiate a change in the delivery of health and social care and housing services by investing a greater budget into telecare technologies. The grant was designed to support vulnerable older people by keeping them safe in their homes and out of hospitals (Audit Commission, 2004).

In 2008, the Department of Health (DOH) introduced their two-year Whole Systems Demonstrators (WSD) Trial Programme, which – with over 6,000 participants selected in three UK sites (National Archives, 2010) – was to be the largest randomised control trial (RCT) of these services in the world. The aim of the trial was to demonstrate the potential benefits of integrated care as supported by telecare and telehealth services. In the UK, older people make up a very high proportion of the population who are in the need of social care services, and many participants of the WSD project were selected from this demographic group as the primary recipients of telecare services.

After the WSD trial took place in the three UK sites, the headline findings for the telehealth programme that were published in 2011 (Department of Health, 2011a) demonstrated that there were reductions observed in mortality rates, emergency admissions, and bed days. However, based on the same success criteria, Steventon et al. (2013) who were involved in the evaluation process, reported that the telecare trial did not cause any major changes in cost, mortality rates, or hospital admissions. Henderson et al. state that evidence on the impact of telecare to support independent living is sparse, and that data on cost-effectiveness is especially limited (2014). Their study demonstrated that telecare was not a cost-effective addition to usual care (Henderson et al., 2014). Overall, WSD results were established to be 'complex' and not compelling by various scholars (Sanders et al., 2012; Cartwright et al., 2013; Henderson et al., 2013, 2014; Roehr, 2013).

In 2013, the Department of Health started planning their second telecare and telehealth initiative, 3millionlives (3ML), in collaboration with the industry, in order to increase the recognition and visibility of these services in England, and thus to "alleviate pressure on long term NHS costs" as well to "improve people's quality of life through better self-care in the home setting" (3ML, 2013). The involvement of a multiplicity of stakeholders in the government's 3ML and similar initiatives implies the "crossing of organizational boundaries, changing structures and shifts in time, as well as roles and potentials for ICTs" (Klecun-Dabrowska and Cornford, 2000).

The provision and use of telecare services are not only limited to large-scale projects like WSD and 3ML, even though these projects have enabled telecare and telehealth technologies to acquire more recognition in communities "against a background of ambition and potential" (Klecun-Dabrowska and Cornford, 2002). Telecare services are provided to older people at their local boroughs and districts. In 2012, approximately 1.7 million people were using telecare services in the UK, yet it was estimated than more than four million people were potential telecare users in England alone (Carers UK, 2012).

Currently, several councils in the UK provide telecare services for their citizens. Telecare systems are not centralised at a national level; a council's own telecare services operate separately from the services in other boroughs, cities, or counties (unless specific partnerships have been created between them). A few examples of local telecare initiatives introduced by the councils are: *Care Connect* by Durham County Council, *Surrey Telecare* by Surrey County Council, *Bristol Careline* by Bristol City Council, *Aberdeenshire Lifeline* by Aberdeenshire Council, and *CareLink Plus* by Brighton & Hove City Council. To access these services, older people are assessed by the social care teams of the councils. Usually, the equipment provided by the council is free; however there is a fee charged for the telecare monitoring services offered, for which the service users are financially assessed by the council.

It has also been more common for the private providers of telecare services, such as the company Telecare Choice, to operate in various areas of the UK. Some councils work together with private service providers or promote private services to their residents. To illustrate, on their official websites, Dorset Council and Leicestershire County Council recommend the services of Telecare Choice as one of the choices for care in the area (Dorset Council, 2019; Leicestershire County Council, 2019). Another kind of partnership that occurs is the agreement made between councils and technology providers, such as Tunstall Healthcare UK.[6] In 2014, Shropshire Council announced that they are committed to working in a collaborative partnership with Tunstall (BBH, 2014); and in 2015, Lancashire County Council appointed Tunstall as a 'development partner' to guide and shape the delivery of adult social care telecare services in the county (Tunstall, 2018). It is evident that such collaborations with industry gathered momentum in past decade.

Sociological and Foucauldian approaches in old age and care research

Evidence-based medicine (EBM), grounded in a positivist perspective, is considered to be equivalent to 'good medicine', and as such, it has been the dominant system of decision-making in healthcare since its initiation in the 1990s (Walsh and Gillett, 2011). The problematisation of evidence in EBM is intended to increase the objectivity of the practices, but it could also obfuscate "the subjective elements that inescapably enter all forms of human inquiry" (Goldenberg, 2006, p. 2626). In most studies conducted in the field of health and social care services, there has been a dominant evidence-based agenda in which quantifiable measures of care are calculated by scholars using economic evaluation models.

The most favoured method of EBM is to use evidence-based randomised control trials (RCTs), which are often referred to as the gold standard of clinical trials. In the RCTs conducted for telecare research, the two main forms of care, (1) traditional care with carer/family support versus (2) telecare, are compared based on the pre-set measures such as: (a) *quality adjusted life year* (QALY), (b) the proportion of individuals admitted to hospitals, (c) the fall rates occurring in different contexts, and (d) the cost-effectiveness of telecare services. QALY is used in cost-utility analysis of interventions, which has its roots in health economics. With similar measures like QALY, health economists seek to assess the value for money of a medical intervention; for instance, the interventions with a lower *cost to QALY saved ratio* are valued more highly than higher ratios. Cost-utility analysis is derived from the archetypal cost-benefit analysis tool. Cost-benefit analysis has been a standard answer to policy problems in the past; it posits universal laws that are claimed to be *value-free* (Goldenberg, 2006). Similar studies that quantify certain aspects of interventions tend to embody an objectivist epistemology that tends to reduce reality into variables in a positivistic and utilitarian manner.

The pressure exerted by authorities to validate certain programmes tends to push forward the need for more quantitative studies with more 'obvious' results. Randomised control trials in particular are seen as the means to this end. The RCT studies conducted in the UK based on the Whole System Demonstrator (WSD) Programme (Steventon et al., 2012, 2013; Cartwright et al., 2013; Henderson et al., 2013, 2014; Hirani et al., 2013;) make use of different theories in data collection, analysis, and interpretations, yet they embody similar comparison methods. Henderson et al.'s (2013, 2014), Steventon et al.'s (2012, 2013), and Hirani et al.'s (2013) studies have a strong focus on quantifiable variables of health and well-being. These include: (a) measures of mortality rates, (b) admission to hospitals, (c) quality of life outcomes, and (d) cost-effectiveness measures. The authors use generically defined, well-established measures of economic theories to carry out their research and contribute to the medical body of knowledge, as well as to policy making. For example, the Department of Health cited a couple of these publications in order to legitimise their next big project, 3millionlives (3ML, 2013), which aims to reach three million people in the UK who are in need of telecare and telehealth services. The government has been criticised for cherry-picking (Greenhalgh, 2012) the results of the studies, pre-dominantly due to differences in telehealth and telecare interventions: whereas the telehealth trial revealed 'positive' findings (based on the pre-determined criteria), the results of the telecare trial were more controversial.

Although systematic review[7] and meta-analysis[8] have been dominant in health and social care research in the UK, there are various studies that focussed on sociological and political perspectives. For example, the alignment of socio-political objectives of the government with economic, social, and personal conduct has been highlighted in the economics literature in the context of technologies and programmes of government, and political rationalities. By *technologies of government*, Miller and Rose (2008, p. 32) refer to "the actual mechanisms through which the authorities of various sorts have sought to shape, normalize and instrumentalise the conduct, thought, decisions and aspirations of others". In the accounting field, Lim (2012) critically examines the government's programmes of old age care and the technologies implemented (both accounting and care technologies). The analysis shows a lack of harmony between the two groups of technologies, and Lim concludes that the 'personalisation' and 'active citizenship' claims do not necessarily lead to greater choice or control over older people's own care (2012).

The government's dominant and official narrative in social services has been shifting towards the use of words such as 'personalisation' and 'putting people first' (Lim, 2012). Carr defines personalisation as

> starting with the individual as a person with strengths and preferences, (...) [with the idea] that people can be responsible for themselves and can make their own decisions about what they require, but that they should also have information and support to enable them to do so.
>
> (Carr, 2008, p. 3)

The vocabulary of personalisation, as built throughout the discourse of personalisation, has been widening to include *personal choice* and *control* as important catchwords. Various policy makers, non-governmental groups and policy implementers are involved in the construction of a framework which aims for an older person to be turned into an empowered individual who is responsible for certain tasks that have been previously recognised as a responsibility of other bodies, or have not been recognised as a responsibility at all. This is referred to as 'responsibilisation' in the governmentality literature (Wakefield and Fleming, 2009; Lim, 2012).

Sorell and Draper's research (2012) studies the debate on whether telecare devices are evidence of a 'surveillance society' or a 'surveillance state' that is developing in the UK. They argue that it is not the intrusiveness on private life or the undesirable paternalism of the telecare services that causes this charge about its Orwellian nature, but that the danger lies where telecare leads to further isolation for the service users. They see it as problematic if these technologies are taken up for the sole purpose of decreasing healthcare spending, and argue that this problem is linked with the eroding welfare state (Sorell and Draper, 2012). There are ways that can more readily address the privacy and independence concerns of telecare users; however, the issues around personal isolation can be more difficult to address. The authors suggest that the notion of independence can be further discussed on the back of policies that support telecare as a *complementary* service, rather than a *replacement* of the care professionals found in the social network of older people (Sorell and Draper, 2012).

It has also been stated that telecare technologies "are first introduced in seemingly benign ways" (Guta et al., 2012, p. 57) and then become the standard by their general deployment. Telecare technologies can cause dangers to those vulnerable people whose "health status locates them at the intersections of medicine, public health, and the law" (Guta et al., 2012, p. 58), such as to those who are living with HIV and individuals with mental illnesses. As the governmental spending on telecare services increase, some concerns are raised about the concept of internalised surveillance through fear becoming a reality. The treatment adherence can quickly become an aspect of the services by reporting on those who 'fail' to adhere to the government-imposed treatments.

In this way, the freedom to choose one's own surveillance (*chosen* versus *imposed* surveillance), as suggested in Sorell and Draper's paper (2012), becomes a 'freedom' that is under question. The technologies that are made acceptable through their productive capacities can, at the same time, become dangerous for those whose identities are stigmatised. Moreover, the freedom to choose, by itself, is stated to be a technique of governmentality that makes the actors accept responsibilities in the form of rational choices. With a lens of Foucauldian scepticism, Guta et al. conclude that telecare technologies might be viewed warily or ambivalently, even deemed to be dangerous due to how the techniques of surveillance will apply to these technologies in the future. Even if certain important needs are met and gaps are filled through their widespread adoption, there is a chance that particular individuals would be targeted more than others.

From an ethical standpoint regarding the future of telecare, Schermer's study on telecare and self-management asks the question: "compliance or concordance?" (2009, p. 690). She identifies two factors that point to a strict enforcement of compliance. First, advancement in technologies will enable more rigorous and pervasive monitoring of health-related behaviours through which the compliance to medically advised lifestyles is monitored, promoted, and enforced. It will become difficult for service users and patients to deviate from regimens, ignore medical advice, or be non-compliant without being noticed. Second is an argument that comes from a 'principle of justice': "Because the society shares the medical costs, patients have a duty to do everything in their power to reduce these costs, and therefore they should be compliant" (Schermer, 2009, p. 690). The normative level of compliance is promoted as a moral good, meaning that people should have a responsibility to live as healthily as possible; otherwise it would be seen as unfair to other people.

Schermer argues that the future use of telecare systems in such compliance-promoting ways can enforce an authoritarian health regime that is legitimised by the morality around distributive justice (Schermer, 2009). To change such a paradigm, it is important to recognise that awareness by telecare developers and medical professionals about the normative ideas of empowerment, concordance, compliance, and self-management plays a role. These normative ideas are embedded in the functionalities of telecare and can be restrictive.

Several Foucauldian gerontological arguments claim that medical power should be regarded as a 'dangerous' extension of power and surveillance that spreads into the lives of older people (Katz, 1996; Biggs and Powell, 1999; Powell and Biggs, 2000; Biggs and Powell, 2001). Powell and Biggs reflect that the increasingly medicalised view of old age is linked with the professional specialisation in bio-medicine, through domination of older people by medical experts (Powell and Biggs, 2000, 2004). Through the use of a Foucauldian narrative, they explore three areas shaped by the self's own consciousness and by medical experts to critically examine the relationship between ageing and self-care. It is concluded that, with the technologies involved in the maintenance of good health, the use of counselling narratives, and bodily enhancement in old age, the existing discourses on the ageing self are overcome or are destabilised (Powell and Biggs, 2004).

The dominance of biomedicine and care technologies creates a dominant narrative of self-responsibility that posits humans as responsible selves (Rose, N., 2001) who look after their own health and social care needs. Powell and Biggs make a critique of the notion 'healthy old age' which is the "result of prudent self-care (...) that one has lived a 'moral life' that has not only its own rewards, but relieves others of any obligation to care" (Powell and Biggs, 2004, p. 20). They continue with the opposite side of this ideal and echo that "becoming unhealthy approximates being undeserving. One is unwell because one is unhealthy, and one is unhealthy because the proper steps of self-care had not been taken in the past" (ibid., p. 20). The notion of self-responsibility therefore can become dangerous when passed through the image of health because it becomes a covert form of moral judgement, on which decisions are based.

On the subject of being responsible for choices, ethnographer Annemarie Mol argues that good care has little to do with the *logic of choice*, in which patients make individual choices that concern their well-being; instead, good care relies on *logic of care* that grows out of collaboration to attune knowledge and technologies to complex bodies and lives (Mol, 2008). Contrary to the *logic of choice*, which gives numerous choices in technologies and treatment plans that individuals can choose from for their own health, Mol argues that the simplistic relationship between a technology choice and its direct consequences is not very representative of the real-world care.

Information Systems (IS) research has been historically adopting sociological approaches. With the assumption that the function of a sociological approach is to reveal social problems and to study the functioning of society, it is applicable for this book to adopt such a lens. My aim is to link the forms of old age construction and its main narratives with telecare technologies, and identify how telecare contributes to this construction process. These narratives are based on normalised forms of certain *ways of being, doing, and speaking* (Foucault, 1969), and certain normalised forms of knowledge and truth. These forms of knowledge and *ways of being* are historically variable, and that a specific version of old age identity is being constituted in the presence of telecare technologies.

Analytical toolbox

The analysis of government publications in this book uses a certain lens that is made up of several analytical tools: critical theory, discourse analysis, genealogical method, and Foucauldian *modes of objectification*, alongside such concepts as discourse, governmentality, identity, and power/knowledge. Telecare information systems (IS) make up a complex system composed of many intertwined technological, political, social, and economic elements. I placed a great emphasis on Foucault's concepts and frameworks due to the applicability of these techniques for historical and genealogical investigation, power and discourse analysis, and formation of subjectivities/identities.

Using a combination of tools, I will investigate: (a) how governments and disciplines study, classify, divide, and regulate old age groups, and (b) how the identity of old age is constituted in ways that are linked with these techniques. These scientific classifications and dividing practices constitute the modes of objectification, which bring forward discussions of power/knowledge and governmentality.

Critical theory

Social scientists associated with the Frankfurt School – such as Habermas, Adorno, Fromm, Marcuse, and Horkheimer – are the originators of the tradition of critical theory. Sometimes referred to as 'critical hermeneutics', critical theory has been characterised as having an emancipatory interest in knowledge (Alvesson and Sköldberg, 2009). The ways in which researchers view social phenomena are open-ended in their historical contexts. Critical theory subjects the ideological and political dimensions of social research, such as asymmetries of power and interests, to deeper analysis and reflection.

With the emergence of the Frankfurt School in the 1930s, positivism and traditional views on science were criticised, and a substantial amount of work was put forward to develop social theories that were politically significant. The Frankfurt School drew attention to contradictions inherent in the functioning of the society, its institutions and modes of thought. The School took Marx, Freud, Weber, Kant, and Hegel as sources of inspiration, and was powerfully influenced by the political environment of Germany and the Soviet Union with the rise of Nazism and Stalinism in the 1930s. Research with psychological depth became more visible. Adorno's and Fromm's work reflected upon the effects of authoritarian upbringing in society, which creates authoritarian relations in the socialisation process and furthers people's compliance with self-subordination (Alvesson and Sköldberg, 2009).

Along with critiquing totalitarian societies, the proponents of this critical theory took commercialisation, mass society, and marketing – guided by technological rationality – as dangers to freedom of thought. Critical theorists reflected that the continuous transformation of people into objects of manipulation makes the subjects vulnerable to control; individuals are in danger of turning into passive, uncritical objects, adapted to mass production and consumption (Alvesson and Sköldberg, 2009). Despite taking a culturally pessimistic view of society, social scientists of the Frankfurt School, such as Habermas, Marcuse, and Fromm, produced work that contains positive, optimistic elements: their critical work studies the possibilities for emancipation from repressive authorities, institutions, and ideologies. Especially after the student rebellion of 1968 in Europe, the works of critical theory – including *An Essay on Liberation* by Marcuse (1969) – focussed on the mobilisation of social forces that enable people to question the dominant social order. This paved the way for marginalised groups who would resist standardisation in later decades; feminists, environmentalists, and, more recently, anti-consumerists, have been the main opposition forces who challenge the dominant logic.

The technocratic ideology of politics uses science and technology administered by experts to solve societal problems (Habermas, 1971). These issues are problematised because the narrow positivist views of science that are utilised in these problem-solving endeavours tend to neglect ethical and political reflections on societal realities. The ways in which experts continuously confront every fragmented part of individuals' lives characterises the human existence with impersonal forces, and can have a destructive effect on the formation of personality. Along with this line of thought, Habermas – unlike members of the early Frankfurt School – states that the legitimation of ideas, traditions, and norms is not only an effect of a dominant ideology; active legitimation happens through the use of argument.

The early critical theory of the Frankfurt School and Habermas's subsequent theory of communication converge at the point of interest in *emancipation*. The tradition of the theory perceives the modern individual to be a manipulated, passive, and objectified unit within the dominance of rationality. Yet it simultaneously depicts the modern individual as having the potential to be autonomous, critical, and self-reflexive. The critiques of technocracy and positivism put forward by several critical theorists are varied in perspective and approach (e.g. Adorno and Horkheimer's polemical style is no equivalent of Habermas's systematisations). Nevertheless, they all share an interest in emancipation, democratisation, and autonomy (Alvesson and Sköldberg, 2009).

Postmodernist approaches in critical information systems research

The study of the role of technology in sociology has been minimal and never a central theme before the rise of the Frankfurt School

(Richardson et al., 2006). In Weberian, Marxist, and Parsonian notions, technology was noted to have an instrumental role to attain an economic end. With the emergence of Frankfurt School ideas, technology became a site for the critique of modernity and was viewed as a tool that is used by the state to subjugate the masses. As it has been argued, the tightly coupled links that build networks between people and things and allow systemisation in modern societies give rise to technical disciplines and hierarchical formations (Feenberg, 2003). The study of control and power are of particular interest here. In later decades of the twentieth century, several sociologists – including Habermas, Bourdieu, and Foucault – developed a more nuanced critique of control, power, and domination, which also expanded the scope of the lens through which the societal role of technology could be studied.

Critical research in the domain of information systems (IS) has been adopted by a growing number of scholars over the past three decades. Creating alternatives to managerialist and functionalist approaches to IS as a reactionary ambition was key in the development of critical approaches (Richardson et al., 2006). Critical theories of technology view technologies as not separate from society, hence from specific political or social systems, and see IS as historically evolving in alignment with other aspects of society (Feenberg, 2003). The application of critical theory in IS asserts an approach which uses the theories that do not solely follow the traditions of the Frankfurt School (Klecun, 2004); the main examples of these theories include: Foucault's genealogy, Derrida's poststructuralist deconstruction, postmodernist interdisciplinary discourse of Lyotard, the social constructivist concepts of Latour, Callon, and Law, and 'late modernity' sociology, such as the work of Giddens (Avgerou, 2000). Therefore, IS research attended the themes of power, domination, conflict, contradictions, and the hidden mechanisms and structures that engender domination (Cecez-Kecmanovic, 2005).

Habermas' work was seen as the most promising in critical IS research in the 1980s, and was compared to the work of his Frankfurt School contemporaries (McGrath, 2005). He worked on the conditions required for ideal speech and refined his methodological approach more comprehensively than his colleagues. However, this methodology was perceived to be inadequate in analysing power relations that were the source of the distorted communications in the first place. Postmodernism adds a sophisticated critique to research by undermining the principle of *emancipation*, and by reflecting on totalising emancipatory discourses. Although it can come in various forms, the central principle of most postmodernist work is *discourse*. Both critical theory and postmodernism fight the claims of objective truth and essentialism with their constructionist stance, while paying attention to the social politics of experience at the local level. History is often emphasised in postmodernist work to analyse how cultural concepts have transformed over time. Postmodernist traditions can be taken up in IS alongside the critical theory for extensive theorisation of power, particularly by focussing on the use of language/discourses.

In the early 2000s, it was recognised that an eclectic critical view, which encompasses Foucauldian ideas, can address power relations, context, and asymmetries in technological innovations on a global scale (Walsham, 2001; Avgerou, 2002; McGrath, 2005). Several pluralistic approaches started emerging out of an amalgamation of critical theory and poststructuralist theories: actor network theory in IS (Klecun, 2004), Critical Discourse Analysis (CDA) (Pozzebon, 2004; Alvarez, 2005), the postmodernist Machiavellian view of power (Silva, 2005), Foucauldian genealogy and his concept of power (Klecun, 2004; Avgerou and McGrath, 2005; Humphreys, 2006; Peszynski and Corbitt, 2006; Willcocks, 2006), the study of Feenberg's postmodernist work (Klecun, 2005), the social shaping of technology, and the social construction of technology (Mitev, 2005).

Feenberg (2003) states that technical codes are biased, dependent on the values of the dominant actors who are involved in the development process of systems. Critical theory of technology mainly seeks for the traces of social bias that show up in various forms of technical rationality through "the social content of technical choices" (Feenberg, 2003). With critical theory, researchers see technologies "not as autonomous but as an instrument of social control placed in the hands of the 'vested interests' which control society" (Klecun-Dabrowska, 2003, p. 39). Critically approaching technologies means that the social values embedded in the design and use of technical systems is investigated to reveal the ambivalent processes between different possibilities. Klecun-Dabrowska reflects that "technology is not a destiny but a scene of struggles" (2003, p. 39). This view summarises the approach of the critical studies in IS.

Klecun's (2005) critical analysis of telehealth IS in the UK within the framework of competing rationalities highlighted and identified two kinds of rationalities: (1) scientific-medical and (2) economic-managerialist. The strongest sign of rationality in medical approaches is that of randomised control trials (RCT), known as the gold standard in evidence-based medicine. Klecun (2005) states that telehealth is societally legitimised through policy documents, more specifically through the image of an 'empowered population'; these national policies embed technical rationality about the IS and portray a simplistic view of the technologies.

Foucauldian research on technologies

Foucauldian approaches have been deployed in IS research, although not widely, yet they have been recognised as a valuable tool. Zuboff's (1988) analysis of the un-neutrality of technology, and Willcocks's (2004) assertion that the behavioural and social technologies are encoded within the material technologies create powerful premises for the use of Foucauldian approaches in the study of IS.

Concepts such as knowledge and power, 'regimes of truth',[9] and the net-like organisation of power and truth can be considered key to Foucauldian research. Brooke (2002) argues that Foucault's power/knowledge can be used to go beyond the Habermasian analyses employed in early critical-theory-influenced IS research. This is where Foucauldian knowledge poses a challenge for the critical theory: it argues that relations of power are not something that one must be emancipated from (Willcocks, 2006). As much as the human subject is placed in relations of signification and production, they are also placed in very complex power relations (Foucault, 1982). The production of knowledge would always be susceptible to the creation of contradictory outcomes between different stakeholder groups. Power is not a relation that is only repressive, but it is also productive; this logic renders the premise of the Frankfurt School's emancipation difficult to implement in research.

Power is internalised and regularised to attain traditional norms in society, and is embedded in routinised, everyday social practices (Silva, 2005). What is integral to the understanding of this disciplinary power is the *panopticon*[10] metaphor that is deeply rooted in normalised practices. In this regard, information technology (IT) can be seen as an electronic panopticon (Zuboff, 1988) through which technological power is internalised. IT in an organisational setting enables the avoidance of in-person contact between employees and managers (e.g. substituted with email communications), while highlighting the work practices through which subordinates can be evaluated by their supervisors, but not vice versa.

Willcocks (2006) reflects that the growth of technological capabilities cannot be disconnected from the intensification of power relations, especially in an era of rising incursion of information and communications technologies (ICTs) into all aspects of life. Foucault may have not privileged material technologies by studying the ICTs directly, but he did privilege the "the behavioural and social technologies encoded and imbedded in material technologies" (Willcocks, 2004, p. 289). With Foucauldian knowledge, we can assert that there is no inevitability/fundamentality that is inherent in the trajectories of technologies in the social world; there exists only the gaps between intentions (Foucault, 1996) as to why and how these technologies are deployed in the way that they are (Willcocks, 2006). This indeterminacy needs to be acknowledged. Things could have been otherwise; no trajectory is "determined by the nature of things" (Hacking, 1999, p. 6). What technology we have now and how it is being used is not something inevitable (Richardson, 2003). The normalisation of workplace practices at an organisation entails the internalisation of certain dominant intentions and logics. Likewise, the development of a particular information system – and the making of the technical code – also reflect the presence of social biases, dominant stakeholder interests, and various paths to discipline.

Discourse analysis

The study of discourses has been a key theme in the social sciences, and discourse analysis (DA) can deepen such study (Alvesson and Sköldberg, 2009). Discourse analysis looks at the construction of reality through language in action. Utterances are context-dependent statements that are meaningful in their private or public settings. This implies that utterances are influenced by what has been said earlier, by the same or by a different person, and hence contain variation. The same phenomenon can be described in different ways by different individuals, and also in different ways by the same individual. Language always presents reality from a specific perspective through these utterances.

Discourse analysis seems to show similarities with poststructuralism in the way that people are taken to be inconsistent, and in the notion that there is an indeterminable gap between a reality out there and the use of language. However, DA differs from poststructuralism with its empiricism and the avoidance of philosophising characteristics of poststructuralism. Nevertheless, DA's use of empirical material does not make it into an approach that uses realist methods, that is, DA is not concerned with finding an underlying reality; the discursive level is its main interest. Discourse, as the object that undergoes discourse analysis, can include kinds of language use, in oral (utterances) and written forms (documents) (Potter and Wetherell, 1987), simply "talk and texts as part of social practices" (Potter, 1996, p. 105). Variations in language use and in accounts of the same event are emphasised, in which language is regarded to be constructive, as well as constructed.

Overall, the empirical materials collected by the researcher – for example, documents – are interpreted on three levels: (1) discursive, (2) ideation, and (3) action and social conditions (Alvesson and Sköldberg, 2009). At the *discursive* level, language does not stand for something else, but only itself, as the object of study. The object of study is merely the language; the states of mind and external conditions are not used for interpretation at this level. However, at the level of *ideation*, the researcher looks at values, beliefs, ideas, meanings, and conceptions for the interpretation of utterances. Finally, at the level of *action and social conditions,* the language and its interpretations are linked to relations, events, social patterns, behaviours, and structures (Alvesson and Sköldberg, 2009). Put simply, this three-layered process starts with descriptions, goes onto interpretations, and then onto explanations; in this way, it moves from the micro textual/discursive level to the macro social level. In this arena, the focus of interpretation is not directed towards straightforward patterns; instead, vagueness, contradictions, and nuances are noted. Inconsistencies and variations become as interesting as consistencies.

Critical discourse analysis

When discourse analysis is undertaken in a critical way, it gains an 'attitude' (van Dijk, 2001, p. 96). CDA looks at the role of discourse in the production and reproduction of power and domination. Fairclough describes CDA's objective as:

> to systematically explore often opaque relationships of causality and determination between (a) discursive practices, events and texts, and (b) wider social and cultural structures, relations and processes; to investigate how such practices, events and texts arise out of and are ideologically shaped by relations of power and struggles over power.
>
> (1995, p. 132)

In the framework of Fairclough, discourse is made up of three dimensions: (1) text, (2) discourse practice, and (3) social practice. According to the model, textual analysis looks at presences as well as absences in texts that are as "significant from the perspective of sociocultural analysis" (Fairclough, 1995, p. 5). This framework can be used to carry out the discourse analysis at the levels of economy (such as of the media), politics (e.g. the characteristics of the market in which the mass media are operating, and their relationship to the state), and culture (e.g. values) (Sheyholislami, 2001). Fairclough's analysis of discourse practice focusses on processes of text production and distribution because "analysis of texts should not be artificially isolated from analysis of institutional and discoursal practices within which texts are embedded" (Fairclough, 1995, p. 9). Social practices imply those hegemonic processes in the institutional or social context in which the discourse partakes; when connected together in a certain way, they establish a social order. Fairclough and Wodak (1997) take language as a social practice and reflect that:

> Describing discourse as a social practice implies a dialectical relationship between a particular discursive event and the situation(s), institution(s) and social structure(s), which frame it: The discursive event is shaped by them, but it also shapes them. That is, discourse is socially constitutive as well as socially conditioned – it constitutes situations, objects of knowledge, and the social identities of and relationship between people and groups of people. It is constitutive both in the sense that it helps to sustain and reproduce the status quo, and in the sense that it contributes to transforming it. Since discourse is so socially consequential, it gives rise to important issues of power.
>
> (p. 258)

We can define social power in terms of discipline and control, and think of power as not being absolute. Specific groups in society may accept, resist, comply with, legitimise, or find such power as natural. The power of dominant groups finds itself in laws, norms, and rules, and is exercised through a variety of taken for granted everyday life actions (van Dijk, 2001).

Fairclough, van Dijk, and other scholars who employ discursive approaches are chiefly concerned with studying language, power, and society. They often use Foucault as an influence in explicitly and implicitly stated ways. Fairclough's approach draws especially heavily upon Foucauldian understandings of discourse, in particular from *The Order of Discourse* lecture by Foucault (1970). It is often not possible to read a literal meaning directly off verbal and visuals signs, and the CDA approach helps to look at those indirect and also absent meanings (Janks, 1997). In Fairclough's version of CDA, the socio-historical conditions that govern the processes through which objects are produced are highlighted. The emphasis on *absent* themes is also another powerful approach. It is fitting to be informed about the principles of certain CDA approaches while approaching the old age topic.

Foucauldian discourse analysis

Foucauldian Discourse Analysis consists of some specific components that are worth being elaborated on. Based on Diaz-Bone et al.'s analysis (2007), the field of Foucauldian discourse analysis is not an internationally integrated field. However, in the studies they have identified that employ the Foucauldian discourse analysis approach, the authors always clarify those key concepts like practices, institutions, power, and subjectivity, almost in an obligatory way (Diaz-Bone et al., 2007).

It is important to point out that Foucault's concept of power does not have a top-down design. Power is not seen to be exclusively located in the state, but it rather is exercised throughout the population, and is present at every level of the social body. Therefore, discourse is not something to be controlled only by privileged groups, even though all forms of power relations refer to the state in certain ways. Nonhoff (2017) states that van Dijk's analyses are mainly centred on actors who have explicit intent to dominate and that his work mostly focusses on dominance and social power that is held by certain groups, elites, or institutions, allowing them to sustain social inequalities. A discourse analysis informed by the Foucauldian notion of power is more conducive to the critical enquiry undertaken in this book.

Sovereign power, which involved a central authority, has been slowly taken over by disciplinary power since the eighteenth century. Foucault argues that modern society is a disciplinary one, in which power is mainly exercised through disciplinary means through a multiplicity of institutions such as schools, prisons, hospitals, etc. (Foucault, 1977). His concept of governmentality involves those techniques that have been designed to govern the conduct of the social body, both at population and individual levels.

Foucault describes *discourse* as a certain 'way of speaking' (Foucault, 1969), and as "historically variable ways of specifying knowledge and truth" (Powell and Biggs, 2003), which function as sets of rules. It refers to those groups of statements that are effective in structuring the way we think about things – how the world is understood – and the ways in which we act on that thinking – how things are done in this world (Rose, G., 2001). Foucault's analysis is concerned with those techniques that make particular ways of doing and speaking normalised. His attention is on the social practices and power relations that give rise to the different institutional regimes, forms of power/knowledge, and logics of subjectification (Foucault 1977; Howarth, 1998). The dual concept of power/knowledge indicates those myriad ways in which mechanisms of power produce different forms of knowledge, and how then this knowledge feeds back into the exercise of power – meaning that they are continuously reinforcing and legitimising each other. This imbrication between knowledge and power is not solely constructed upon the notion that "all knowledge is discursive and all discourse is saturated with power" (Rose, G., 2001, p. 138), but, more importantly, it indicates that the most powerful discourses – in terms of their social effects – depend on the claims and assumptions that their knowledge is true.

For Foucault, discontinuities and continuities in history reflect the fact that things are no longer perceived, classified, and known in the same way as before (Foucault, 1994b). For him, discourses are discontinuous practices; however, some of the discourse would be continuous over time, until society establishes the new form of truth based on the steady accumulation of knowledge. Overlaps, disruptions, and discontinuities occur with the reconfiguration of this new norm/rationality/truth. Foucault's genealogical method is concerned with the "historical limits and conditions" of discourses, which have the capacity to "direct and distort the personal and institutional narratives that can subsist within them" (Biggs and Powell, 2001, p. 6).

Foucault states that "it is not enough to say that the subject is constituted in a symbolic system. It is not just in the play of the symbolic that the subject is constituted. It is constituted in real practices – historically analyzable practices" (Foucault, 1997, p. 227; Olssen, 2014, p. 34). Another argument of Foucault establishes that "there is nothing to be gained from describing this autonomous layer of discourses unless one can relate it to other layers, practices, institutions, social relations, political relations, and so on. It is that relationship which has always intrigued me" (Foucault, 1967, p. 284; O'Farrell, 2005, p. 80). This marks the recognition of other objects than discourse, although their relationship with the discourse is primary. It is important to highlight that Foucault avoided the traditional idealist/materialist division or cause and effect relations in his work. We cannot divide the history into "two levels, the airy level of ideas (or discourses) and the earthy and 'real' level of 'material' occurrences" (O'Farrell, 2005, p. 81). For example, economics does not constitute the material infrastructure; and theory the frivolous superstructure; or that an idea does not cause a social event to occur, or vice-versa.

One of the material components of the discursive system is the telecare technology and their practice in connection with older people. My focus in this book is not to detect the coercive ways with which the government is implementing their IT strategies; the emphasis is rather on those discourses that are formed through various power/knowledge mechanisms of governmentality. It is important to pay attention to those old age discourses that might be enacted or undergoing changes in a new *context*, in the presence of telecare technologies.

The Foucauldian toolbox

Foucauldian thinking is concerned with the historicity of the link between power and knowledge, and evidently how certain strata in society came to be as they are. Versions of postmodernism, critical theory, and hermeneutics are encompassed by Foucault's writings. His power analysis and discourse analysis are distinct in their capacity to avoid objectivistic claims about the world (Alvesson and Sköldberg, 2009).

Foucault's work contributes to the analysis of old age in the following ways: first, his analysis of disciplinary techniques, as well as his analysis on the relationship between madness and medicine, have parallels with the societal perceptions of old age and older people. In his work, he describes "how the 'elderly', 'criminals', and the 'mentally ill' are constructed through disciplinary techniques such as the 'gaze'" (Powell and Biggs, 2000, p. 6). Second, the historical critique approach of Foucault enables the destabilisation of taken for granted assumptions about ageing, and helps to diagnose current social arrangements (Powell and Biggs, 2003). And finally, Foucault's approach makes it possible to analyse both the discourses embodied in social policies and those functioning within society.

Foucault worked on diverse topics and problematised such issues as deviance, madness, illness, criminality, and sexuality (1967, 1977, 1980a). Because these issues are conceptualised as socially constructed problems, Foucault in return has problematised "the role of the 'expert', social institutions, social practices and subjectivity that seem 'empowering' but are contingent socio-historical constructions and products of power and domination" (Powell and Biggs, 2000, p. 6). His theories are relevant to old age because he recognises that social practices "define a certain pattern of 'normalization'" (Foucault, 1977, p. 72). These social practices are mediated by 'experts', such as managers, who interpret older people through a process of 'assessment'. Care managers can be seen as one part of the panoptic technology (Foucault, 1977) who scrutinise and normalise judgement on older people through several discourses, such as older people as service users, as clients, or as consumers. Because the ageing bodies and individuals are located in a network of normalising discourses, the power relations in this political field aim to render ageing individuals as docile as well as productive subjects (Smart, 1985).

Powell and Biggs (2003) reflect on the methodological tools of archaeology and genealogy as fundamental to Foucauldian research. They are key in the investigation of social aspects of ageing because they can be used "to disrupt history at the same time as giving history a power/knowledge reconfiguration" (Powell and Biggs, 2003, p. 1). Archaeology includes the systematic method of investigating and tracing statements in the historical archive, such as official statements and policy documents (Powell and Biggs, 2000). Genealogy, on the other hand, puts archaeology to practical use, links historical data to the current context, and investigates *discontinuities*. Through this investigation, the ways in which human beings are made subjects by power/knowledge practices are revealed.

The genealogical method

In its approach to discourse, genealogy distinguishes itself from archaeology because it focusses on the study of processes within the web of discourse (Powell and Biggs, 2003). With a genealogical approach, researchers can look at which discontinuities and continuities exist in a given context (Powell and Biggs, 2001). Discontinuities and inconsistencies have been a part of Foucault's work in which the origins of discourses were tracked in the form of *epistemes* – "the ordered fields of knowledge (...) which are common to the discourse of a whole epoch" (Alvesson and Sköldberg, 2009, p. 250). In Foucault's own words, genealogy is

> a form of history which can account for the constitution of knowledges, discourses, domains of objects, etc., without having to make reference to a subject which is either transcendental in relation to the field of events or runs in its empty sameness throughout the course of history.
>
> (Rabinow, 1984, p. 59)

By getting rid of the subject itself as an analysis theme, the historical – and contextual – constitution of the subject can be accounted for by the genealogical analysis.

"Genealogy", as Foucault states,

> does not pretend to go back in time to restore an unbroken continuity that operates beyond the dispersion of forgotten things; its duty is not to demonstrate that the past actively exists in the present (...) Genealogy does not resemble the evolution of a species and does not map the destiny of a people. (...) it is to identify the accidents, the minute deviations - or conversely, the complete reversals - the errors, the false appraisals, and the faulty calculations that gave birth to those things that continue to exist and

have value for us; it is to discover that truth or being does not lie at the root of what we know and what we are, but the exteriority of accidents.

(Rabinow, 1984, p. 81)

The genealogical method looks at the power relations through oppositions to the power strategies; for example, investigating 'insanity' to find out what is meant by 'sanity' in society, or how the field of 'illegality' creates the meaning for 'legality' (Foucault, 1982).

Foucault used discourse to analyse diversity in configurations, assumptions, claims, categories, and so on; it is a logic of reasoning that permeates the social world, and forms its objects systematically, rather than being a mere use of language in social contexts. Foucault's interest lies in the constitution of objects and subjects through discourse. This why 'power' has always been present in Foucault's work. It was at first subjugated to discourse analysis, and later was subordinated to genealogical methodology. In genealogy, the origins of discourses, as well as their regularities, randomness and discontinuities, are studied. Foucault's work started with its archaeological phase that studied the forms of discourses with isolated discursive descriptions. It continued with a genealogical phase that studied origins of discourses, incorporating a critical engagement with power. In the first period, the archaeological method was used to disregard statements of truth, map out systems of thinking, and write a history of the present. The archaeological approach can be seen as a method through which to manage and organise forms of knowledge and determine similarities and differences among them. Similarly, the genealogical method uses the same substrata of knowledge; however, the object of interest sways from the silos of knowledge to the mechanisms of power, which have historically provided the grounds for the construction of certain dichotomies – such as normal and deviant, true and false, and so on (O'Farrell, 2007). For this to be achieved, Foucault looked at non-discursive practices in addition to the discursive ones, such social institutions as sexuality, prison, psychiatry, and so on.

Foucault offers a different way from the Frankfurt School in investigating the relations between rationalisation and power. In the construction of 'power', Foucault disregards the use of conventional concepts – such as ideologies, structures, individuals, etc. – as well as any definition or abstraction of power. Foucault's disinterest in 'who possesses power' creates an understanding of power that is unlocalised and changeable, and, in theory, everywhere. There is no clear theoretical formulation of power by Foucault, as a theoretical order would have delimited or defined power.

Therefore, it would be proper to say that power is a mode of action upon actions; that power relations are rooted in the social networks of the society; and that power relations are not constituted above the societal level. It would be an abstraction to suggest an existence of a society without power relations; to be a part of a society makes the mode of action upon actions an ongoing process. This is precisely why the analysis of power relations in a given society is politically critical of their history and of the conditions necessary to transform (and abolish) some actions (Foucault, 1982).

'The genealogy of the modern subject' (Rabinow, 1984, p. 7) looks at and analyses the parts of discourses and practices that deal with knowledge, power, and the subject. Studying the problematisations of the subject, of power/knowledge, and of government aligns with the general aim of Foucault. This aim has been to discover the points in history at which particular practices were moulded into reflective techniques, and at which points particular discourses emerged out of these techniques, and were rationalised to reflect objective truths. For example, Powell and Biggs's study states that genealogy of old age disrupts narratives of 'choice' – the language that has been embedded in social care policy in the UK (Powell and Biggs, 2000).

The next sections focus on the construction of subjectivities and identities, modes of objectification, bio-power, and governmentality to further understand the elements of the genealogy of the modern subject.

Subjectivity, identity, and human kinds

Subjectivity can be demarcated as a core concept to understand ageing (Powell and Biggs, 2004). Foucault's work focusses on subjects that are "caught in various webs of discipline, power and modes of liberation" (Katz, 1996), and asserts that "subjectivity itself must be denounced as a principle of domination" (Dews, 1984). The Marxist philosopher Althusser's positional subjectivity asserts that we live in a concrete world as well as a symbolic one in which "we pattern our subjective experiences in ways that reproduce concrete relations" (Katz, 1996, p. 11). For Foucault, the material manifestations of subjectivity represent an aspect of reality that is systematically formulated by discourses. In the Foucauldian analyses of micro-levels of culture, local politics, and marginalised groups, one can find rich discursive, social and historical layers wherein relations of power and knowledge outlie the processes of economic exploitation and labour.

Individual subjects are both social agents and social constructions. Foucault states that

> it may be that the problem about the self does not have to do with discovering what it is, but maybe has to do with discovering that the self is nothing more than a correlate of technology built into our history.
>
> (Foucault, 1993, p. 222)

The organising of social relations is mediated through the potential of a belief/category; the more idealised this belief/category is, the greater its potential. For example, 'the aged' is a subject category, a category of social construction, which becomes meaningful through relations of power with the articulation of self-reinforcing institutions, practices, and ideologies (Riley, 1988). Dominant ideologies secure their hegemony in a context-dependent way. In the temporality of ideologies and subjects, the same ideology can both operate to secure or resist the hegemony, and the same subject to embody both resisting and dominant strategies. This asserts that no one subject position or no system of meaning (ideology) can stay permanently in power (Katz, 1996).

The production of subjectivity within normalising environments, such as clinics, is the exploration arena for Foucauldian analyses. One concept that is visible in the scholarly discussions of subjectivities is *identity*, such as the ageing identity that is used in this book. Concepts of subjectivity and identity are sometimes used interchangeably, although their differences are highlighted in some studies. It can be said that identity has its roots in the modernist tradition, whereas subjectivity is founded on post-structuralist and postmodernist thought, and focusses on the making of the subject and the making of identity. To conceptualise the relation between subjectivity and identity, cultural theorist Weedon offers a definition:

> Identity is perhaps best understood as a limited and temporary fixing for the individual of a particular mode of subjectivity as apparently what one is. One of the key ideological roles of identity is to curtail the plural possibilities of subjectivity inherent in the wider discursive field and to give individuals a singular sense of who they are and where they belong.
>
> (2004, p. 19)

For example, 'assessment' can be considered a central technique that makes an individual into an old age object of power/knowledge

(Foucault, 1977). In assessments, an ageing body is established in relation to normalised standards of risks, which render older people as objects of economic, social, and psychological narratives that address 'frailty', 'financial resources', and required levels of 'supervision' (Powell and Biggs, 2000). This

> indicates the appearance of a new modality of power in which each individual receives as his status his own individuality, and in which he is linked by his status to the features, the measurements, the gaps, the 'marks' that characterise him and makes him a 'case'.
> (Foucault, 1977, p. 192)

To illustrate a point, older people are socially positioned in specific ways and this positioning creates a particular identity. This identity that older people occupy is actively constructed in discursive contexts, such as through national policies. Identities in general are constructed through public discourse, and they occur in association with each other, including age, gender, race, sexuality, disability status, etc. Although, in a particular context, certain identities are prioritised (Fealy et al., 2012); the social care policies generate a context in which the identity of old age has been foregrounded.

Older people are constructed as a particular social category (NCPOP, 2009); the identity of old age arises from the categorical label 'old age', which "might appear natural and obvious" (NCPOP, 2009, p. 8). However, this categorical label is "contingent, unstable and the product of particular historical circumstances" (Ainsworth and Hardy, 2007, p. 269). The social construction of older people is often with reference to the utilisation of health and social care services, and therefore an identity of dependency is constructed through this (Ainsworth and Hardy, 2007; NCPOP, 2009).

The creation of identities constitutes a complex process in which power and subjectification overlap. The sociologists Dagg and Haugaard (2016) analyse this complex process through Foucault's work, 'The Subject and Power' (1982), in which he elaborates on the relationship between the creation of social subject and power:

> This form of power applies itself to immediate everyday life which categorizes the individual, marks him by his own individuality, attaches him to his own identity, imposes a law of truth on him which he must recognize and which others have to recognize in him. It's a form of power which makes individuals subjects. There are two meanings of the word subject: subject to someone

else by control and dependence, and tied to his own identity by a conscience or self-knowledge. Both meanings suggest a form of power which subjugates and makes subject to.

(1982, p. 212)

In this quote, Foucault argues that subjectification constitutes a process that categorises the individual; the individual becomes a carrier of meaning (Dagg and Haugaard, 2016). With this, the individuality of the person is marked, giving them a particular identity, a particular way of being. This identity does not only socially position the person for others, but also constitutes an own sense of identity. However, this is not an arbitrary social construction, but a representation of the regime of truth,[11] the truth that highlights the normalising effect of all discourses. Through this social construction, an interactive process is formed in which the individual recognises their position as perceived by others; "in this act of recognition they become subject to someone else's normalising judgement, which constitutes a form of dependence upon another as a validator of that subject identity and, consequently, that other imposes upon them a form of control" (Dagg and Haugaard, 2016, p. 397). This 'external validation' becomes a form of self-knowledge and comes to define the individual's perception of self. In other words, the individual becomes both a subject and an object of knowledge. As an object, they are subjected to the evaluation of others, and this establishes their subject position in society (Dagg and Haugaard, 2016).

The elements of this external knowledge formation form the basis of this book. Although the creation of a social subject happens through a complex system of power and subjectification processes, the aim here is to focus on those practices of power/knowledge that constitute a form of dependence upon individuals as a validator, and impose upon them a form of control. Therefore, from this point on, the construct of *old age identity* in this book will refer to an *abstraction of an old age identity*, which is represented through the medium of telecare policies. I intently define *identity* to comprise the power/knowledge formations that impose a form of control structure upon old age subjects. The public texts reveal explicit and implicit ways of positioning older people that bestow on them particular old age identities.

The construct of *identity* also resembles the concept of *human kind*. Philosopher Ian Hacking introduces the mechanism of *looping effects* in his discussion of human kind, which details the iterative processes between knowledge production on objects and formation of self-knowledge (1995, 1999). He draws inspiration from Foucault in relation to the production of knowledge. Hacking's *human kinds* (1995) – or *interactive kinds* (Hacking, 1999) – means "kinds about which we would like to have systematic, general, and accurate knowledge; classifications that could be used to formulate general truths about people; generalizations sufficiently strong that they seem like laws about people, their actions, or their sentiments" (Hacking, 1995, p. 352). The conceptualisation of a human kind, as opposed to natural kinds, assumes that a human kind primarily classifies people and their behaviour.

Social sciences classify the interactive kinds (Hacking, 1999). Calling the *person A* with the *human kind H* may make the society treat A differently, as much as making a difference to A because the human kind H would possibly be loaded with moral connotations. Creating kinds to classify people affects how individuals think of themselves, their self-worth, and how they remember their past too. This is how a 'looping effect' is generated, because people of a certain human kind behave differently, and the kind changes constantly. Each change creates a new field of causal knowledge for the sciences, wherein the old knowledge about the kind is updated. This new way of sorting again changes the behaviour and self-conception of the people classified; "kinds are modified, revised classifications are formed, and the classified change again, loop upon loop" (Hacking, 1995, p. 370). It is not the case that wholly new human kinds are devised continuously; rather, it is about the reorganisation: building on the old kinds.

There is a regular tendency to strip human kinds of this value/moral content by biologising and medicalising them as part of the instrumental human sciences, which are named by Hacking as "the great stabilizers of the Western post-manufacturing welfare state" (Hacking, 1995, p. 364). The studies conducted in human and social sciences to detect law-like regularities generate acceptance, intervention, and consensus, thereby becoming what we take the knowledge to be, and forming the system of government. As part of this system of governing, oftentimes the causal connections between kinds are taken to be more comprehensible at a biological level, as opposed to the connections operating at a social or psychological level (Hacking, 1995). The word *biological* stands for "biochemical, neurological, electrical, mechanical, or whatever is the preferred model of efficient causation in a given scientific community or era" (Hacking, 1995, p. 372).

The concept of identity resembles the concept of a human kind. In a way, by theorising the concept of human kind, Hacking creates a nuanced version of identity, in terms of the iterative processes between external and internal knowledge formations. The ageing identity, which is central to this book, also undergoes looping effects; therefore it is inevitably a human kind. The reason why this concept is important is because the identity formation does not occur either just by external (to the individual) knowledge formation or just by self-knowledge. It is still essential to be reminded that the knowledge itself is not just the product of the state. The social positioning of a certain *kind* of people through governmental policies can generate looping effects. This is because people classified interact with the classifications, and thus, by implication we have all the more reason to reveal these classifications.

Modes of objectification

As subject-constructing disciplines, gerontology and old age studies provide an arena for the exploration of the use of modes of objectification. The three modes of objectification that transform humans into subjects were studied in 'The Subject and Power' (Foucault, 1982). These are (1) the processes "that categorize, distribute, and manipulate; [2] those through which we have come to understand ourselves scientifically; [3] those that we have used to form ourselves into meaning-giving selves" (Rabinow, 1984, p. 12). These three modes of objectification can be referred to as: (1) *scientific classification*, (2) *dividing practices*, and (3) *self-subjectification*. The first mode is the mode of enquiry and of *scientific classification*, which is reflected on the status of sciences. The second mode, *dividing practices*, divides the subjects either within themselves or divided from others. The example of objectivising the subject as 'mad' versus 'sane', or 'sick' versus 'healthy' belongs under this mode of objectification. The third mode studies *self-subjectification* – the process of a human being turning themselves into a subject.

Scientific classification practices transform people into kinds of subjects and have been used as invaluable techniques for the production of knowledge in the human sciences: for example, in disciplines such as sociology, psychiatry, and criminology. These practices offer ways to study, organise, define, and codify human attributes based on the grand categories of the *normal* and the *deviant/pathological*. Foucault's *The Order of Things* (1994b) studies the production of subjects as objects of knowledge. It asserts that the Renaissance's *epistemes*[12] of the enlightenment later developed into scientific discourses of the West. Examples include the objectification of the speaking subject in linguistics; "of the subject who labours, in the analysis of wealth and of economics"; and "of the sheer fact of being alive, in natural history or biology" (Foucault, 1982, p. 777). One of these subject positions is the aged subject. In the same tradition as in other human sciences, the sciences of geriatrics and gerontology that arose in the late nineteenth century produced new knowledge based on this new subject.

Maintaining social stability by separating, categorising, normalising, and institutionalising populations entails the use of *dividing practices*. Historic examples include the segregation of lepers from the non-diseased, the mad from the sane, and the criminals from the good people. The rise of psychiatry in modern times and its application in prisons, hospitals, and clinics is another example of dividing practices in action, as well as the modern process of stigmatisation, regularisation, and medicalisation of sexuality mainly in Europe. The rise of modern programmes of rehabilitation and reform, and the convergence of liberal humanism with disciplinarity, gave space for the birth of the prison (Foucault, 1977). With dividing practices, the subjects are given a social and personal identity by which they are socially objectivised and categorised. Exclusion through scientific mediation is the main mode of manipulation of the dividing practices through which groups are formed and given an identity. Put simply, this mode looks at how institutions objectify human subjects.

The coexistence of *classification* and *dividing practices* entails that, while professions study and classify groups, the governments and institutions discipline, divide, and regulate these groups. The mode of subjectification by which a person turns themselves into a subject, *self-subjectification*, includes *technologies of the self* –

> techniques that permit individuals to affect, by their own means, a certain number of operations on their own bodies, their own souls, their own thoughts, their own conduct, and this is in a manner so as to transform themselves, modify themselves, and attain a certain state of perfection, happiness, purity, supernatural power.
> (Foucault and Sennett, 1982)

For example, the discourses of sex, as part of self-understanding, gained momentum in the nineteenth century; it was followed by an obsession around sexuality, own health, and the growth of medicalised discourses of sexuality (Rabinow, 1984). The study of technologies of self in *The History of Sexuality* (Foucault 1985, 1986) reflects the idea that one's ideas about oneself are merely the recurring consequences of the self-subjectification practices of Western society. Classification and dividing practices, when combined with self-subjectification practices, construct modern subjects. To continue with the example of sexuality: human sciences classify problems and experiences of sexualised subjects, the systems of power stratify and institutionalise the kinds of sexual subjects, and the *technologies of the self* give reflexive means to individuals to problematise their sexualities. Dividing practices and subjectification can be combined to analyse the historic processes; however these two modes are still distinguishable on the analytical level.

When applied to the study of old age, this theoretical framework focusses on the analyses of the techniques that are used to problematise ageing subjects, rather than focussing on the conventional formulations and analyses of ageing. In the example of old age, three technologies have been identified through which the ageing self has been reshaped by medical experts (technologies for self) and by the self's own consciousness (technologies of self): (1) good health management, (2) bodily enhancement, and (3) the use of counselling narratives (Powell and Biggs, 2004).

This book takes *scientific classifications* and *dividing practices* (two of the modes) as the basis of analysis, through which conclusions can be drawn on old age identity. This is largely because my principal investigation is about how governments and disciplines classify, study, divide, and regulate old age groups. Therefore, the 'technologies of regulation and collective control' (Powell and Biggs, 2000) will be given a preference, and the construction of old age identity will be investigated through the lens of public policies. Policies form discursive systems of power/knowledge through which discourses are enacted and normalised. Revealing the explicit and implicit ways in which they position older people will outline a constructed old age identity.

Governmentality and bio-power

Since the rise of the state in the sixteenth century, a new political structure and form of power developed. Pastoral power, a power technique originating from Christian institutions, is a historical predecessor to the regime of bio-power. The element of individuality, which serves a function in religious institutionalisation, has come to be part of pastoral power and of the modern state in its new form. The *state* is therefore manifested through a new kind of pastoral power and modern individualisation techniques (Foucault, 1982). As opposed to the religious expression of salvation – which relates to a different world – the modern version of salvation manifests through well-being, security, health, etc.

What marks the beginning of the era of bio-power is a collection of techniques that can achieve the control of the population and of the body; the development of disciplines, universities, schools, and the emergence of research and policies regarding public health, birth rate, housing, and migration. Bio-power mechanisms heavily depend on explicit calculations; categories such as species, population, and fertility become "the object of systematic, sustained political attention and intervention" (Rabinow, 1984, p. 17). Government and medicine became components of the medico-administrative regime that resulted from the eighteenth- to the nineteenth-century health crises. The spread of normative rationality of bio-power reinforced the reliance on statistical methods and judgements that divide the population into healthy and unhealthy, normal and pathological, and living and dying to calculate and monitor the health of the population. The apparatuses of normalisation make possible the normalisation of the law through the addition of principles of psychiatry, medicine, and social sciences as part of legal discussions. "The law operates more and more as a norm, and (...) is increasingly incorporated into a continuum of apparatuses (medical, administrative, and so on) whose functions are for the most part regulatory" (Foucault, 1980a, p. 144).

Bio-power enables the policies to have an impact on biological health, and it enables the state to govern individuals by influencing their biological frameworks. For example, the aged body became the centre of social and scientific discourses on old age in the nineteenth century. Through the disciplining of aged bodies, the disciplining of knowledge about old age was made possible. Technologies of bio-power come together and make the objectification of the body possible. The disciplinary technologies in diverse institutional settings – such as in schools, hospitals, prisons, etc. – aim to create docile bodies through different methods. Training of the body, standardisation of actions, and control of the space enforces continuous disciplining and supervision to enable certain objectives in those settings. These objectives could include facilitating productivity in a factory, ensuring orderly behaviour in a school, and controlling epidemic diseases in a population (Rabinow, 1984).

Foucault's notion of "power in knowledge" (Deetz, 1992, p. 77) emphasises the inseparability of the concepts of power and knowledge. The intimate relationship between the development or deployment of specific knowledge and the exercise of power is formed through classifying, measuring, calculating, and standardising in institutionally controlled environments. While knowledge makes possible the exercise of power, this exercise in turn also creates knowledge, in its both repressive and progressive forms.

Political rationality lies at the centre of disciplining and regulating, which binds the subject and power together. The most popular example as given by Foucault to represent a framework of a disciplinary technology is the aforementioned model of the *panopticon*, as devised by Bentham in the late eighteenth century. Besides being a model of functioning, the panopticon organises spatial arrangements and humans in particular ways as a visual cue to the functioning of power. The rationality behind the panoptic model could, at first, be predicted to be that of productivity and efficiency; yet the aspect of normalisation is the key. Norms organise, and they are also the results of controlled orderings around which individuals are systematically distributed. This normative ordering forms the key component of *biopower*, the regime of power by the state, in the form of a government that is concerned with fostering life and the care of the population by measuring, qualifying, hierarchising, and distributing around the norm. Human sciences that regulate and create, directly or indirectly, the modern body serve as the knowledge base for the exercise of disciplinary bio-power.

The notion of *government* does not only refer to the management of the state or to political structures, but rather a designation to direct by which the conduct of individuals is made possible (Foucault, 1982). The specific forms of government in a given society are manifold in the way that they overlap, cross, cancel one out, and reinforce each other. In modern societies, the state does not pose as only one form of exercise of power any longer; rather, all other forms of power relations do refer to it in a certain way. When these power relations come under further state control, they are increasingly "governmentalized, that is to say, elaborated, rationalized, and centralized in the form of, or under the auspices of, state institutions" (Foucault, 1982, p. 793). For example, the *governmentalisation of living* has been progressively happening through the contribution of a series of new scales, such as the measure of quality-adjusted life-year (QALY). This type of governmentalisation makes "social and personal consequences of living with disease (...) an object of political concern", and the living "knowable, calculable and thereby amenable to various strategies of intervention" (Wahlberg and Rose, 2015, p. 1).

The study of the body through advanced information technologies that enable scanning, mapping, imaging, etc. has provided ways to categorise and make visible functional and dysfunctional conditions (Rabinow, 1996; Katz and Marshall, 2004). Functional measurements are made transparent through technologies and flow with ease between bodies, individuals, and populations. Unlike in the historical binary of the normal/pathological in medical sciences, the dysfunctional states in postmodernity can be adjusted and enhanced through therapy, experiments, lifestyle, diet, and drugs. This situation enables the creation of a web of data that connects scientific and online communities, population statistics, research studies, and marketing. What comes next after the transparency and visibility of functional/dysfunctional states is the development of bio-identities that rely on these states – 'biological citizenship' (Rose and Novas, 2005). People know themselves based on the ways their biosocial lives are deemed worthy; their biology becomes improvable and manipulable. Bio-citizenry embraces an element of curiosity by the individuals about life choices and decisions, besides the larger mobilisation of lobbies and groups around the issues of pharmacological research, reproductive rights, health, and environment (Katz, 2010).

Foucault's specific interest was in neoliberalism as a form of governmentality because of the ways in which it involves individuals in the process of governing, and how this governing becomes embodied. Neoliberalism emphasises the dominant doctrine since the 1970s that takes market exchange as a guide for all human action. It reconstructs the state's powers by minimising economic interventions by the state, and by diminishing the obligations to provide for the welfare of its citizens (Harvey, 2007). This means fewer social services provided by the state, and wider privatisation in these services. Rose and Fukuyama use Foucault's governmentality to explain processes of neoliberal economics today, and study how neoliberalism's main function is to self-govern (Fukuyama, 1996; Rose, 1999). This is because the individuals are in charge of their own access to social services rather than the government providing these services for them. Neoliberalism's continuous efforts to shrink state services require individuals to manage their own access to social services (Maskovsky, 2000). Therefore, the governmentalisation of the state is principally about "the continual definition and redefinition of what is within the competence of the state and what is not" (Foucault, 1991, p. 103).

Problematising all power/knowledge relationships was a consciously taken decision by Foucault. He described his own position to be, not one of apathy, but of "hyper and pessimistic activism" (Rabinow, 1984, p. 343). With his interest in micro resistance, Foucault states that "everything is dangerous, which is not exactly the same as bad. (...) I think that the ethico-political choice we have to make every day is to determine which is the main danger" (Rabinow, 1984, p. 343). This reflects the importance of trying to observe and resist the main danger in any specific time and context, and "to choose the least dangerous of several dangerous alternatives" (Alvesson and Sköldberg, 2009, p. 258). The activism in Foucault's work is not linked with attacking institutions or persons; the main objective is rather to question a technique, a form of power. In a series of oppositions to the power of men over women, psychiatry over people with mental illness, medicine over population, etc., the struggle is not for or against the individual, but rather against the "government of individualisation"[13] (Foucault, 1982, p. 781), and against the privileges of knowledge. This government of individualisation categorises the individual, attaches them to an identity, and imposes a law which they themselves and others must recognise in them. Put simply, this technique makes individuals subjects.

Because power is intricately intertwined with knowledge, Foucauldian thinking asserts that there is no 'innocent' knowledge, and it dismantles the notion of neutral, rational, and progressive research. The knowledge that comes with emancipatory claims can also contribute to certain forms of subjectivity due to defining the conceptions and the ideals of its claims that are linked with 'normality'. Even progressive poststructuralist research can include a dimension of power that creates a desirable state of subjectivity and is deemed more playful and fluid; nevertheless, the monitoring and normalisation processes might still be in play in those researches, only in a more flexible form (Alvesson and Sköldberg, 2009).

Key remarks

The creation of 'old age' as a separate group in the UK appeared as a product of the late nineteenth century. Old age became recognised as a social issue in the early 1900s, one that needed attention with new social policies. It was mainly constructed around poverty and dependency until the post-war welfare state era in the 1940s. Along with the establishment of the NHS, the modern government took the central responsibility over older people through developing a moral framework. The construction of ageing went on to gain more nuances over time.

The idea of 'active retirement' emerged, and, in the 1980s, themes of youthful retirement, fulfilment in life, and active lifestyles became a part of the understanding of ageing. Thus, with the 'modernisation of ageing', old age in late modernity took on a different meaning. But in the 1990s, when anxieties around the equitability of the welfare state arose due to a series of financial constraints, old age started to be seen as an economic burden on the state. These uncertainties destabilised 'old age' by transforming the institutions – such as welfare, retirement, and family – through which older people's identities have been defined. Because the crisis of old age is increasingly associated with the ways in which individuals – rather than society as a whole – handle the demands of ageing, the 'moral framework' of the state has been shifting to a completely new domain.

This domain has been defined by the principles of postmodernity, in which traditional structures – such as trade unions, class, and the welfare state – are being abandoned. People are increasingly put into the position of holding responsibility for negotiating their lifestyles and making their own choices about how they want to conduct their lives. Linked to this, increasing levels of separation between government and the services that the government funds have created a so-called 'hollow state'[14] (Estes and Linkins, 1997), which has been observed since the late 1980s. The period during which the private spending in health and social care services has increased in the UK coincides with the period of growing societal anxieties about the future of the provision of services by the state.

The making of the aged body and the older population into the central focus of scientific knowledge and political practices has its origins in the period during which age became a regulatory theme in family, schooling, work, and retirement. The existing discourses of old age are, therefore, products of the ways bodies and populations have been historically problematised through the regulation of age. These narratives can be subsumed under three overarching categories:

1   The medicalisation of old age
2   Older people as new group of consumers
3   The association between old age and social welfare

As aforementioned, the provision of telecare services is predominantly for the use of older people. Due to the challenges presented by ageing populations and the increasing demand on health and social care services, technological care has seen a global rise lately. In the past decade, the UK Government has been consistently advocating the widespread adoption of telecare services, and the technology industry has been presenting new technological innovations to enhance well-being and health as the population ages. On the back of these changes, telecare information systems occupy a greater part of public social care policies, and thus they create a new domain in which the old age narratives can find their place. This is because information systems (IS) form an organised system through which the collection, storage, organisation, and communication of information takes place. Older people are the primary actors of telecare information systems who interact with technologies and other telecare actors, and are processed, interpreted, classified, and organised within this system.

The practices of legitimising telecare services and the process of handling information about older people via telecare technologies entail the knowledge of what is known about old age and ageing. This knowledge is embedded in policies, institutional practices, and the functionalities of telecare, in various ways. In the next chapter, I will investigate the enactments and redefinitions of this knowledge, in the form of discourses of old age, in relation to telecare technologies.

The following list covers key concepts and constructs that were highlighted in this chapter.

Table 2.1 List of key concepts and constructs

Concept/construct	Definition
Discourse	A historically variable yet certain in context way of speaking or writing to specify how things are and how they are done.
Dividing practices	The mode that divides the subjects, either within themselves or from others, through such processes as: regularisation, medicalisation, and exclusion through scientific mediation; the means through which institutions objectify the human subjects.
Governmentalisation/ Governmentality	The way in which the state exercises control over bodies and the population. It also refers to the way in which people are taught to govern themselves, through shifting power from a centralised authority – like a state or institution – and dispersing it among a population (MedAnth, 2010).
Grand discourse	The overarching narrative that comprises multiple and distinct perspectives, usually continuous over a specific time frame.
Human kind	Group of people about whom we have systematic and general knowledge through law-like generalisations about them, their actions, or sentiments.
Identity	A limited and temporary fixing for the individual. In this book, identity refers to the abstraction of an identity, normalised and represented through policies.
Normalisation	Construction of an idealised norm of conduct; the processes through which ideas and practices become taken for granted.
Old age	There is no definite biological stage for old age. The most common form of referring to old age is on the basis of chronological age. However, this is a normalised construction, because 'old age' as a categorical label appears natural and obvious (NCPOP, 2009). The construction of old age varies culturally and historically; the pension age (65 years in the UK in 2019) is usually the threshold for old age for governmental and administrative purposes.
Power	A repressive and productive relation that is omnipresent in all levels of social relations. Each type of power – such as sovereign, pastoral, and disciplinary power – consists of a "particular set of techniques, rationalities and practices designed to govern or guide people's conduct" (O'Farrell, 2007).
Power/knowledge	Mechanisms of power produce knowledge by collecting information on the activities and existence of individuals. These types of knowledge reinforce further exercises of power and further knowledge gathering.
Scientific classification	The ways to study, organise, define, and codify human attributes based on grand categories of the *normal* and the *deviant/pathological*, often using the status of sciences and financial justifications.

In light of the history of old age and its connections with telecare, we can divide the initial query "How is the identity of old age constituted in relation to telecare technologies?" into three refined questions:

Q1: Through which scientific classification practices do old age discourses surface in relation to telecare?
Q2: Through which dividing practices do old age discourses surface in relation to telecare?
Q3: How do social care policies enact and transform the grand narratives and the identity of old age?

Mapping out the scientific classifications and dividing practices will elaborate on the language that produces knowledge, enacts certain discourses, and socially positions individuals in certain ways. Then, the ageing discourses enacted and generated in relation to telecare will be linked to the current constructed identity of old age.

Notes

1. Indexation is when income payments are adjusted by means of a price index, which adjusts to inflation. Deindexation is when wages are no longer index-linked.
2. Young and middle-aged population supporting older citizens.
3. Medical gaze refers to "discourses, languages, and ways of seeing that shape the understanding of aging, and (...) increase the power of, the health professions" (Biggs and Powell, 2001, p. 95).
4. After Jean-François Lyotard published his Postmodern Condition, there has been an ongoing discussion on the notion of modernity. Bonacker (2006) states that "in this debate one can find several descriptions for the current changes of modernity: modernity today means 'postmodernity' (Lyotard, 1984), 'multiple modernities' (Eisenstadt, 2000), 'second or reflexive modernity' (Beck, Giddens & Lash, 1994) or 'liquid modernity' (Bauman, 2000)" (p. 73).
5. The systematic description of diseases.
6. A technology company specialising in digital health and care solutions, mainly in telecare and telehealth.
7. "A systematic review answers a defined research question by collecting and summarising all empirical evidence that fits pre-specified eligibility criteria" (CCACE, 2011).
8. "A meta-analysis is the use of statistical methods to summarise the results of these studies" (CCACE, 2011).
9. Regimes of truth are "socially constructed power-constituted determination of what is rational" (Avgerou and McGrath, 2005).
10. Panopticon is a type of prison architecture planned by the British philosopher and social reformer Jeremy Bentham during the industrial revolution. The aim of the architecture was to implement a system of surveillance over

the prisoners, and its design included a tower in the centre encircled by a building of cells that accommodate prisoners all of which face the tower. This system allows permanent surveillance and a state of consciousness of the inmates, even when a guard is not present in the tower. The result is the creation of disciplinary power.

11 Foucault describes regime of truth as follows:

> Each society has its regime of truth, its 'general politics' of truth: that is, the types of discourse which it accepts and makes function as true; the mechanisms and instances which enable one to distinguish true and false statements, the means by which each is sanctioned; the techniques and procedures accorded value in the acquisition of truth; the status of those who are charged with saying what counts as true.
> (Foucault, 1980b, p.131)

12 "I would define the episteme retrospectively as the strategic apparatus which permits of separating out from among all the statements which are possible those that will be acceptable within, I won't say a scientific theory, but a field of scientificity, and which it is possible to say are true or false. The episteme is the 'apparatus' which makes possible the separation, not of the true from the false, but of what may from what may not be characterised as scientific" (Foucault, 1980b, p. 197).

13 "Everything which separates the individual, breaks his links with others, splits up community life, forces the individual back on himself, and ties him to his own identity in a constraining way" (Foucault, 1982, p. 781).

14 The hollow state typically contracts outs its provision to private sector and keeps for itself the monitoring and inspection responsibilities (Estes and Linkins, 1997).

3 A critical enquiry into discourses and the identity of old age

This chapter provides background information by describing the National Health Service (NHS), social care services under the NHS, and the national telecare policies linked to social care services. While doing this, some attention will be given to the privatisation of the NHS services and the implications of the budget cuts on different segments of the population, such as older people. Documents used to provide a descriptive account of NHS in this section (i.e. the government papers, policies, industry reports, etc.) are purposefully selected as they are related to and are the products of the history – especially the fiscal history – of the NHS.

Finding themes in the analysis necessitates the use of the history of telecare services in relation to social care services and in relation to NHS. Therefore, particular attention will be given to the political landscape, as it is inextricably linked with the production of policy solutions in social care services. Descriptions will focus on components of telecare policies that generate or sustain the narratives around old age. The thematisation process in this chapter is informed primarily by Foucauldian Discourse Analysis (FDA) and some principles from Fairclough's (1995) approach to Critical Discourse Analysis (CDA). I will thematise the documents in the following order: (1) policy analysis through forewords and (2) policy analysis through visual elements.

NHS and social care services

The NHS was born out of a 1930s vision that was put forward by the Socialist Medical Association and then proposed by the Labour government in 1948. Under the umbrella of this new institution, the nationalisation of UK hospitals became the priority. As a product of a twentieth century post-war social policy, the NHS was set up on the basis of medical need, rather than the ability to pay. This was a historically important moment, especially for low-income class people and the more vulnerable groups in the population. This universal, equitable, and free health service meant that the healthcare services would be funded through general taxation.

The NHS was (and continues to be) supported by the Department of Health in England, the Scottish Executive Department of Health in Scotland, the NHS Directorate in Wales, and the Department of Health, Social Services, and Public Safety in Northern Ireland (House of Commons Library, 2012). Each country within the UK chose to structure its own health service in different ways.[1] Nevertheless, across the board, the NHS continued to be kept as the universal free health service by successive governments since its inception. When it was created, several associations that had provided medical insurance before the establishment of the NHS joined forces to create the British United Provident Association (BUPA). Although in later years BUPA gained a monopoly in the provision of private medical insurance, the formation of the NHS pushed private healthcare to the margins of the system in the UK. As the largest employer in Europe, the NHS was providing healthcare services cheaply to the public, and it was very popular amongst the population.

The economic crises of the 1970s and underfunding of the services by successive governments challenged the smooth running of the NHS. With the emergence of neoliberal ideologies and the principles of free market that came with them in the 1970s–1980s (Harvey, 2007), new sub-disciplines – such as health economics – became more prominent in the development of principles that concern efficiency within the NHS. When the Conservative leader, Margaret Thatcher, came to power in 1979, such free market principles and assumptions only became more prominent. The Thatcher era saw the introduction of strict anti-union and anti-strike legislations in the 1980s. These effectively entailed the weakening of strong trade unions, of which the employees of the NHS (including non-medical staff) had been a part. It also saw the implementation of public sector reforms with business principles onto the welfare state (History and Policy, 2007). These changes paved the way for the successive privatisations of the NHS by the governments of Major, Blair, Brown, and Cameron (Scott-Samuel et al., 2014). Thus, in the last few decades, a move towards a market-based healthcare system has been observed. Several changes took place during and after the Thatcher years, such as the annual increase in prescription charges (Scottish Parliament, 2013) and, more significantly, the shifting of responsibility for the provision of long-term care for older people from the NHS onto the local authorities (Scott-Samuel et al., 2014).

60 A critical enquiry into old age

With the financial squeeze of the NHS in the late 1980s, the scope of services was reduced first by shifting the long-term care responsibilities of people with mental illness to local authorities. This led to the selling and privatisation of mental health facilities and wards (Open Democracy, 2014). Local authorities were also obliged to pay for private nursing homes for the long-term care of older people. Although the NHS was still publicly popular, the number of people with private insurance had substantially increased in number since the 1980s (Commission on the Future of Health and Social Care in England, 2014). This coincided with the expansion of global private healthcare corporations, which had become popularised in Europe.

With growing concerns about the understaffed condition of the NHS in the 1990s, the NHS was taken on the path of a 'third way' by Tony Blair and New Labour. This 'third way' project was concerned with the modernisation of the NHS to make the services attractive to the public again. This was presented with a view that positioned patients as 'consumers' who are given choices by healthcare professionals. With its consumer-centric principles, this vision to modernise the NHS was thereby echoing business-centric privatisation. Before Blair's extra funding pledge for the NHS (Watt, 2000), the New Labour[2] government were working collaboratively with Private Financial Initiatives (PFIs) to open new hospitals.

PFIs, which were introduced during the Conservative government of Major in 1992, soon became the principal funding bodies for the hospital building programme of the government (Shaw, 2010). PFIs meant that public-private partnerships were being formed through which public infrastructures were funded with private capital. The use of PFIs was limited until 1997, when the Exchequer announced the fiscal policy of reducing government debt, and the government needed to be financed by the private sector. The use of PFIs became even more wide-spread when the Labour Party's Health Secretary announced that year, "when there is a limited amount of public-sector capital available, as there is, it's PFI or bust" (Physicians for a National Health Program, 2007).

In 2000, the responsibility of commissioning healthcare for patients was given to the NHS bodies called Primary Care[3] Trusts (PCTs). PCTs could buy hospital care for patients from private healthcare providers. In 2003, the Health and Social Care Act passed, which provided the basis for a radical transformation in the NHS by giving importance to Hospital Trusts. With the economic growth of the 2000s, more than 100,000 new nurses and doctors were recruited (LSE News, 2011), and the NHS went through its largest hospital-building programme (Secretary of State for Health, 2000). With PFIs, the private sector had power over the management of NHS, due to owning and maintaining several NHS hospitals.

All these changes made to the NHS by New Labour were based on the need for additional capacity. However, by the middle of the 2000s, marketisation enabled the private sector to be competitors against the public provision of healthcare (BBC News, 2005). After the general election in 2005, several policy changes took place that reflected a shifting rationale and a move towards the creation of a market in healthcare. Buzzwords, in the policies of later years, changed to include terms such as 'patient choice', 'competition', 'improved efficiency', etc. (Department of Health, 2010a, 2010b, HM Government, 2009, 2010). The NHS reform that created a market in the provision of secondary care[4] gradually shifted towards an increasing involvement of the private sector in primary care.

In 2006, the first contract was signed with the private health and social care company Care UK to set up a general practice (GP) and walk-in centre in Dagenham, London (Care UK, 2017). The government continued to encourage more companies to take over general practices or set up new centres due to a shortage of practices in certain areas. The opening of private practices/polyclinics was extended to the country as a whole. In 2008, NHS London instructed PCTs in London to open a centre led by GPs and/or a polyclinic in their area (Londonwide Local Medical Committees, 2008). This was a step to consolidate small GP surgeries into clinics with more GPs that would provide some services already provided at hospitals. While this step was taken to provide more personalised services for the patients due to being closer to their homes, the decision created the means for corporations to be able to invest in these local clinics.

With the 2007 financial crisis, The Conservative Party popularised the need for an austerity programme in the UK based on considerations about past government expenditures. The programme was initialised by the elected coalition in 2010. That year, the ideal of a regulated market was followed through by the Conservative Party-led government. The Health and Social Care Bill submitted in early 2011 by the Secretary of State for Health proposed to abolish the control structures that New Labour had put in action over the healthcare market and privatisation. The Primary Care Trusts (PCTs) were to be abolished (they were abolished in 2013), and the powers of the Department of Health and the Secretary of State with regard to the provision of universal health service were also to be reduced following the bill (Department of Health, 2011b). The time frame for the austerity policy had been drafted to be five years; however, the Conservative leader, David Cameron, announced that the public spending reductions were going to continue until further stated. At the beginning of 2017, new public budget plans were put forward along with the Conservative Party's manifesto that included a pledge to end the deficit by the middle of the 2020s (Reuters UK, 2017). However, based on the Institute for Fiscal Studies' (IFS) analysis, it has been forecasted that a third parliament of austerity is awaiting Britain after 2020 (IFS, 2017).

The UK's government austerity programme has brought significant changes to the ways in which public services are organised and operate. For example, reductions to the number of staff in public services has increased workloads for remaining staff, limited the time of frontline staff for public-facing work, and reduced the number of staff in operational roles such as social work. An increased tendency has also been observed for one service to pass cases on to another service, and some specialist staff have withdrawn from services. It was stated that, due to resource constraints, staff were more prone to define responsibilities of their service more narrowly, and third-sector organisations have had to fill in gaps in council service more frequently, despite their own funding reductions (Hastings et al., 2015). Councils have had to make small changes to a range of services, such as cutting on opening hours of libraries and leisure centres and reducing the frequency of street cleanings (Hastings et al., 2015).

These public service cuts go hand in hand with objectives to privatise certain services. In this regard, the case of the NHS continues to be a long and frequently debated one that has been under much public scrutiny. In 2016, the Government announced that they would sell off the majority of shares to the private sector with the aim of "creating a profitable business model" (UK Parliament, 2016). With this, public investments into the NHS were put on hold, and the NHS was driven towards a regulated market system.

Unlike the provision of health services through the NHS, social care services historically have not been free at the point of delivery in England. Local authority support is means-tested (as will be explained below), and those individuals who receive funding are still expected to contribute their income towards the cost of their care (Jarrett, 2017). Since 1997, there have been policy proposals of successive governments about how individuals should pay for their social care. Most recently, pledges were made towards the betterment of social care services while Conservative governments were in power. The two most recent Conservative leaders, David Cameron and Theresa May, both pledged to cap the overall social care costs (Department of Health, 2017); however hitherto these pledges were not actualised.

These proposed changes were related to the two kinds of measures that affect how the care of older people is funded: (1) *care caps* and (2) *means tests*. A *care cap* indicates that individuals will not pay any more for their care needs once they meet a certain limit. The £72,000 care cap was proposed during Cameron's government (2010–2016), and was planned to be introduced in 2016; however, the government has deferred it at least until April 2020. The second parameter that determines the funding of care is the *means test*; it assesses an individual's assets and finances, and a decision is made as to how much they should contribute towards their own care. In the current system, older people who have assets worth more than £23,250 do not receive any support from councils, meaning that many individuals end up with a burden of care costs. Only savings and capital below £14,250 make an individual eligible to be fully funded by the local authority, and an amount between £14,250 and £23,250 means that the local authority pays for some part of the individual's care, based on a sliding scale. As with the proposed care cap changes, the changes to means tested benefits were planned to come into effect in 2016 but have also been postponed. In this deferred plan, the £23,250 upper limit was set to be raised to £118,000, and the £14,250 lower limit was set to be raised to £17,000 (Age UK, 2017).

It is worth noting that during the introduction of these proposals, some changes were made as to how the means tests would be calculated. Even though the limit has been proposed to be raised to £118,000, this amount was planned to include the value of the individual's house, as opposed to the current system where "the value of a person's home is only counted in this limit if they are in residential care or nursing homes" (Full Fact, 2017). The manifesto of the Conservative Party puts residential care and home care means-testing on an equal basis. This change in the testing poses significant risks to some people who are receiving care not in a residential care home, but in their own home, because they might lose eligibility for care due to these changes. It has been estimated that "out of those in their 70s who would get support at home if they needed it under current rules, an estimated 12% to 17% wouldn't be eligible under the rules proposed in the manifesto according to the IFS", because their homes will be taken into account (Full Fact, 2017). These changes have been reported in the media under the title 'dementia tax' even though the term is not a new one. The Alzheimer's Society describes dementia tax as: "People with dementia face the highest costs of care of any group and have to pay the most towards their care. This is why charging for care is described as 'The Dementia Tax'" (Alzheimer Society, 2011). According to the statistics given in the 2013 report of the UK Homecare Association (UKHCA), around 60% of people who receive care at home have dementia (Roberts, 2013). The proposed changes in the means testing would inevitably affect mainly older people, and those with dementia even more so.

During the austerity period, further social care saving plans worth £824m were put forward by the government for the 2017–2018 period. The Association of Directors of Adult Social Services reported that "total cumulative savings in adult social care since 2010 will amount to over £6bn by the end of March 2018" (Adass, 2017, p. 4), meaning that local authorities have spent significantly less on social care between 2010 and 2018 than they did in 2010, when austerity began. It has also been reported that the spending cuts in all public services have affected mostly women, people of colour, and the working class, implying that at the intersection of these three identities, there lies triple discrimination through gender, race, and class (Women's Budget Group, 2016). The austerity measures in social care services had detrimental effects on certain minority groups of the population, such as older people, more than others.

According to the comprehensive study of Loopstra et al. (2016), support for poorer older people has significantly declined, creating rises in death rates amongst the people aged 85 and over. It has been also stated that "the number of people getting state-funded help has plummeted by at least 25 per cent" (King's Fund and Nuffield Trust, 2016, p. 6) from "over 1.1 million in 2009 to 853,615 in 2013/14" (King's Fund and Nuffield Trust, 2016, p. 15). A report by London School of Economics reflects that half a million older and disabled people who would have received social care in 2009, received no local support in 2013 (Fernandez et al., 2013). Therefore, the cuts in healthcare and social care services have affected many individuals, in particular older people. The reducing level of spending on these services has also been linked to a stagnating rise in life expectancy in the UK since 2010 (Marmot, 2017).

The creation and amendment of social care service policies exemplified in this section mediate and lead to changes in the provision of telecare services in direct and indirect ways. Telecare services have been part of governmental agenda and national policy papers, and they have been introduced in the form of local telecare initiatives with collaborative work of the NHS, Department of Health, and local authorities. Political interest in the promotion of telecare services has been reported to be due to: (1) changes in the ageing demographic; (2) increased pressures on health and social care services; (3) technological advancements; and, especially, (4) the shrinking budgets of health and social care services (Department of Health, 2010a, 2010b; Mort et al., 2013). Care from home is being promoted as an appropriate solution to these changes.

Policies and information strategies relevant to telecare services

The 1990s saw an increasing number of studies presenting research about older people and care technologies. These studies provided the grounds for the government to increase their publications on these topics. A housing research report published in 1994 by the Department of Environment (whose current equivalent is the Department for Communities and Local Government) emphasised that the responsibilities of supporting older people have been moved from institutions to the communities, and older people are becoming more consumerist, seeking choice and independence (McCafferty, 1994). The study also showed that four in five older homeowners desired to stay in their homes independently. The Royal Commission on Long Term Care[5] recognised the importance of modern technologies for their potential in improving the lifestyle of older people in imaginative and profitable ways (Royal Commission on Long Term Care, 1999).

During the late 1990s, the older people's charity Age Concern[6] was involved in the debate of ageing and plotted the demographic change that awaits the UK: in 1995 there were less than nine million people aged over 65; it was forecasted that, by 2030, there would be 50% more older people (Age Concern, 1998). When the NHS began, life expectancy in the UK was around 50 years, and 60% of the population was under 20. However, in the late 1990s, life expectancy increased to 80, and 50% of the population was estimated to be over the age of 50 in subsequent decades (Age Concern, 1998). Although this was a success of improved social conditions and medicine, healthcare costs for older people were found to be significantly higher than those of other age groups (Ermisch, 1990, p. 42; Anchor Trust, 1999). An increase in the number of older people was therefore an indicator that healthcare costs would also increase.

In the late 1990s, the UK government directed its initiatives towards promoting health and independence, modernising care services, and delivering value for money (Department of Health, 1998). With these ideas, telecare services emerged in a network of information systems. While enabling older people to live safely and independently in their homes, telecare strategies were expected to be aligned with a wide range of healthcare, social care, and housing-related government initiatives.

With the recognition of various technologies in the information strategy white paper, *Information for Health* (NHS Executive – DOH, 1998), the government was setting national strategies for the local implementation of various services. These involved technologies such as electronic patient records, the NHS Direct telephone and online information services, telemedicine, telecare, the NHS net network between hospitals and GP surgeries, and information systems linking GPs and community pharmacists. The government was determined to invest in telecare technologies at a national level, as these services were seen to have a key role in the government's plans to modernise the NHS. After this white paper, the nationwide development and application of telecare was given a higher priority.

The Department of Health's *Modernising Social Services* white paper in 1998 (Department of Health, 1998) identified various failures and problems in social care services. These issues were linked to a low level of public confidence in social services, and a call for *modernisation* was emphasised. This modernisation entails a support for people's independence, welfare reforms, and social inclusion. The protection of vulnerable individuals, particularly older people, is in the foreground of the paper. With this white paper, clearer responsibilities for local government were identified by the central government, and new targets for quality and efficiency were set for the councils. The Social Services Modernisation Fund that was introduced via this paper was made up of a £1.3 billion budget to be spent over three years on various projects that promoted independence. *Modernising Social Services* is an influential paper that restructured social services, improved joint working between healthcare and social care, and provided the grounds upon which the Care Standards Act 2000 was built.

Some telecare initiatives were trialled in the late 1990s, and these gained momentum with broader governmental recognition. The Lifestyle Monitoring Telecare System was one of the most notable examples. It was the result of a two-year project funded by the Housing Corporation's[7] Innovation and Good Practice (IGP) grant[8] and by British Telecom (BT). The project was trialled by BT and Anchor Trust[9] in designated homes located in Newcastle, Ipswich, Liverpool, and Nottingham. The aim was not to create a finished product; rather, it was to learn the issues that must be addressed in order to offer successful products to older people, that is, products they can benefit from to remain independent (Anchor Trust, 1999). The system proved to be a prototype for telecare solutions in the upcoming years.

This monitoring telecare system was designed to work without a need for community alarm equipment or a wearable physical device.

It recorded daily activity patterns via passive infra-red (PIR) movement sensors, magnetic proximity switches, and temperature sensors in various rooms. The sensors were located with wireless communication, and the user had the choice to turn the system on and off by dialling a designated number. The data gathered through the telephone network was then sent to BT laboratories for analysis. Once a normal pattern profile had been created for each person on the trial, the system was looking for deviations from this pattern. If any deviations occurred, an alert call would be generated. Upon answering the phone, the user was asked to press 2 for assistance, or 1 if they felt that no assistance was required. As an escalation step, a nominated carer would be called if 2 was pressed by the user or if the alert call was not answered. Blue light services were not yet integrated into the network at this point as the trial was not a large-scale one. After the trial, focus groups, in-depth questionnaires, and interviews with users were undertaken to record experiences and expectations. The independent evaluation done by the Institute of Human Ageing at the University of Liverpool pointed to the success of the trial, with high satisfaction rates from older people and their carers (Anchor Trust, 1999).

Various councils continued working together with BT to deliver telecare services in their areas. Several other trials were taking place simultaneously during this time, and the number of initiatives was increasing. With regard to the former, the joint venture named Liverpool Telecare Pilot was formed by Liverpool City Council in 2004. With regard to the latter, an initiative called Better Government for Older People (BGOP) was set up by the government in 1998 as a partnership between the public, private, and voluntary sectors. The key partners of the BGOP were older people, and the initiative aimed to shape policy and decision-making at both local and national governance levels. Older people (which were then defined as those aged 50 and above) supervised research projects until the end of the initiative when the projects were completed. However, soon after the end of the initiative, it was turned into a *Network* with the addition of 350 local member organisations to share good practice, and "to bridge the gap between the policy intentions of local and central government" (Community Care, 2002). The network is partly funded by the government, and partly by its subscribers. The BGOP also funds the Older People's Advisory Group (OPAG), an offshoot launched in 1999 that aims to influence local and national policy. OPAGs still exist today in various counties and councils, and they do local work.

In 2000, *The NHS Plan* was presented to the parliament by the Secretary of State for Health. The problem it addressed was defined as (p. 12): "old people falling in the cracks between the two services" (social care and healthcare), and the solution it offered was to ensure that resources would be shared between the NHS and social services for the first time in the NHS' history (Secretary of State for Health, 2000). New care trusts were introduced with this plan to commission healthcare and social care services under the same organisation. This bill prioritised getting support for people at risk to remain independent at home, as well as securing their safety and security. They also started the debate about a need for new technologies for the independent living of older people and people with disabilities. The modernisation of IT systems and placement of extra funding into information technologies were on the government's agenda in the years following the bill. It was claimed that 50% more people would benefit from assistive technologies[10] and community equipment services. These ranged from basic care equipment, such as grab rails, to more sophisticated devices, such as fall alarms.

In 2001, the Department of Health issued a strategic framework document about older people's housing (Department of Health and DETR, 2001b) that gave special emphasis to older people's specific needs, including the use of new technologies to support their independent living. Due to a change in the ageing profile, the provision of affordable and appropriate housing for older people was impacted in various ways. The report's aim was to encourage and enable local authorities, including the local NHS and councils, to (a) reflect upon their strategies for the community, (b) improve services, and (c) help organisations that provide housing and services to ensure that their services are accessible to older people. Technology was put in the heart of the housing talks. Contributing factors for this focus were: the increased use of technology in people's daily lives, the emphasis on preventative services that can help to support older people in their own homes, and the healthcare costs of an ageing society. At this point, community alarm technologies were being used by many older people; however, a drawback of these systems was the need for the user to initiate the call. New technologies such as telecare were deemed by the government to be more preventative in their approach, hence offering benefits for older people.

In 2004, the government announced their plans to invest £80 million over the period of 2006–2008, in what they named the *Preventative Technology Grant*. The purpose was: "to initiate a change in the design and delivery of health, social care and housing services and prevention strategies to enhance and maintain the well-being and independence of individuals" (Department of Health, 2005b, p. 8). This change involved substantial investments in telecare technologies. The grant was designed to support vulnerable older people by keeping them safe in their homes and out of hospital (Audit Commission, 2004).

Consecutive national publications about telecare followed: *Strategic Business Case Models for Telecare*; *Building Telecare in England*; and *Independence, Well-being and Choice* by the Department of Health (2005a, 2005b, 2005c), and *Telecare Implementation Guide* by the Care Services Improvement Partnership (CSIP, 2005) – the partnership that operated between 2005 and 2008 under the Department of Health to support the local delivery of health and social care policy. The papers included: finances, advice, implementation guidelines, ethics, and performance assessment guidelines of telecare services. This furthered the case for telecare technologies as a national panacea in the form of prevention, enablement, and early intervention services.

With the publication of the white paper, *Our Health, Our Care, Our Say: A New Direction for Community Services* (Department of Health, 2006), some concerns were put forward regarding old age and disabilities in the population. It was estimated that over two-thirds of NHS activity and an estimated 80% of costs are linked with one-third of the population who are over 85 years old and/or have severe disabilities. To overcome this problem, the Department of Health was intending to increase the joint commissioning between primary care trusts and local authorities for better service integration, rather than providing fragmented services. Future objectives of this paper were to increase the choices given to patients and to extend support for people with long-term needs to live independently, with special emphasis placed upon assistive technologies. The government was invested in demonstrating whether technologies such as telecare benefit or enhance the quality of life (QoL) of individuals and of their carers, and whether they deliver gains in the cost-effectiveness of care. To reform health and social care services as a whole, the government also expressed determination to tackle care inequalities

> (...) across social class and income groups, between different parts of the country and within communities. The new emphasis on prevention will help close the health gap; so will encouraging GPs and other providers to expand services in poorer communities.
> (Department of Health, 2006)

Expanding services meant that telecare was also to be extended beyond the small-scale trials to all communities of the country.

70　*A critical enquiry into old age*

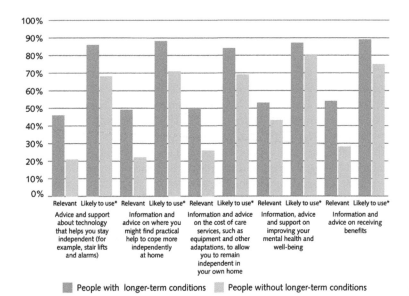

Source: *Your health, your care, your say* questionnaire
N = 25,666 then weighted for population
* Total out of those who said it was relevant

Figure 3.1 Responses to the question "Services that could be made available – which are relevant to you and which would you use?" from people with and without longer-term conditions. People with longer-term conditions, including a large proportion of older people, find the use of assistive technologies more than twice as relevant as people without longer-term conditions. The image is from the Department of Health's 'Our Health, Our Care, Our Say: A New Direction for Community Services' white paper (2006, p. 118). Licensed under the Open Government Licence for Public Sector Information v3.0- http://www.nationalarchives.gov.uk/doc/open-government-licence/version/3/.

The circular from the Office of the Deputy Prime Minister (2006), which was supported by the Department of Health's *Building Telecare in England* paper, aimed for fair allocation of the Preventative Technology Grant. Based on the strategy, this fund was to be allocated within two years and amongst all councils in England who were responsible for their community's social services. The government recognised the effectiveness of telecare only as an integrated service with many partners; it expected councils to work with others – such as the NHS, housing authorities, voluntary sectors, service users, carers, etc. – in developing telecare services.

With the introduction of subsequent government reports on the future of social care (HM Government, 2007, 2009), care discussions were more focussed on older people, independent living, prevention, and telecare. Initiatives were introduced in 2009, such as the Older People's Prevention Package, to encourage the use of prevention services by older people. Care guidance on telecare services was also part of the package. At around the same time, the Department of Health introduced their two-year Whole Systems Demonstrators (WSD) Trial Programme, the largest randomised control trial (RCT) of telecare and telehealth services to date. With over 6,000 participants selected in three UK sites (National Archives, 2010), they aimed to close the evidence gap around the effectiveness of telecare and telehealth technologies, and to demonstrate the potential benefits of integrated care.

With the announcement of social care-related Department of Health papers within a short period in 2010 (Department of Health, 2010a, 2010b; HM Government, 2010), the vision of individuals with more control over their own care was introduced. After the restructuration of how services were to be commissioned, local social care services – including telecare – became a bigger part of the councils' responsibilities. The role of the government shifted towards facilitating the changes, rather than being directly involved; it was a shift towards less top-down and more local accountability. The councils were now held to account by the local communities for the services they provide and the experiences of service users. The Adult Social Care[11] teams in the councils had certain responsibilities, such as providing information and advice to local citizens, enabling and improving the local preventative and early intervention care services, and working in close partnership with housing authorities and the NHS (Department of Health, 2010a).

These publications also discussed the topic of funding options. It was stated that an unfair situation was arising between generations because "the majority of people to benefit from a fully tax-funded system would be older people, and yet it is working-age adults who would face the largest burden in paying for it" (HM Government, 2010, p. 128). The case was supported with statistics from the Office for National Statistics that stated that the people aged between 65 and 74 were one of the wealthiest age groups in Britain, and that by contrast young people had debts from student loans and mortgages. In this way, the financial justifications for telecare were put forward through the government's publications.

As the years have passed, Telecare initiatives have become a bigger part of the Department of Health's and councils' agenda in searching

72 *A critical enquiry into old age*

for more cost-effective ways of caring for older people and people with complex long-term conditions (Sanders et al., 2012). After the results of the WSD programme were released in 2012, and were deemed to be effective by the government, the Department of Health quickly started a new initiative called 3millionlives (3ML). DH believed that "at least three million people with long term conditions and/or social care needs could benefit from the use of telehealth and telecare services" (3ML, 2012). The government aimed to use this campaign as an encouraging example for greater use of remote monitoring ICTs in health and social care (HM Government, 2015).

3ML was a national call for the authorities to work together with the private sector over the next five years in the development of a market for telecare services. Department of Health was aiming to create an environment to encourage the uptake of telecare services by rewarding organisations for adopting these technologies. Along with other trade associations, the Telecare Services Association (TSA)[12] supported and funded this project, which is the main telecare accreditation body in the UK that has been publicly endorsed by the government. After this point, social care and NHS services started working more closely with industry. Telecare services were expected to bring about major implications for health and social care services by transforming the order of care and extending the reach of healthcare outside of the consulting rooms and hospitals (Oudshoorn, 2011). Following the governmental push by the telecare trials, initiatives, and changes in commissioning structures, there were various pilot projects launched at local councils across the country – including notable projects in London, Surrey, Durham, and a few others – conducted by the social services of the related councils.

Thematising policies

Publicly available information and guidance documents by the UK government, policy papers (white and green papers), and social care related industry and research reports are the main sources of information used for analysis. Health and social care publications of the NHS, UK Government, Department of Health, and of industry bodies in England were systematically searched, and the documents that incorporated information on care in old age and/or care technologies were chosen.

The most relevant 40 documents mainly consisted of government publications, aimed to inform the public and the industry. Seven of them were selected that could be representative, content-wise, for the rest of the documents. One commonality between the selected publications was the presence of a foreword at the beginning, which was intended to present a condensed version of the document, usually written with the personal voice of a politician. First, the sentences in which a recurring and/or an interesting theme was observed were copied off from the text. Then these sentences were given codes with such keywords as 'choice', 'control over own care', 'dependence', 'independence', 'locality', 'modernisation', 'use of statistical data', and so on. Based on the rate of occurrence, interrelatedness and the thought-provoking value of these codes, the clusters were grouped into overarching groups, with each group incorporating a set of interrelated themes.

In addition to the forewords, a combination of over 20 illustrations, diagrams, case descriptions, and quote bubbles were used from 13 white papers, green papers, guidance documents, flyers, and easy-read government documents, which are part of the initial 40 documents in the pool. The purpose is to investigate whether the graphics carry the meanings attached to key themes, and to identify emerging new themes, if any, in addition to those obtained through the thematisation of forewords. The assumption is that the graphics and other forms of non-textual information operate through a visual method rather than a textual/verbal one, because "very often visuals and 'verbals' operate in a mutually reinforcing way" (Fairclough, 1989, p. 28). The end purpose is to concretise and expand those themes that have been identified in the foreword coding.

Studying the problematisations of the subject, of power/knowledge, and of governmentalisation aims to discover points in time during which particular discourses have emerged, been reinforced by techniques of government, and been rationalised to reflect "objective" truths. The presence of telecare technologies creates a new context in which these discourses and the identity of old age can potentially undergo changes in terms of being expanded or transformed. The modes of dividing practices, scientific classifications, and technologies of self in the regime of bio-power explain the techniques by which people are turned into objects and subjects of dominant discourses. Two of the modes, namely scientific classifications and dividing practices, form the basis of analysis. The practices of self-subjectification (the third mode of objectification) involve perceptions, experiences, and everyday practices of older people, as this mode is concerned with the creation of subjectivity by people's own means. As in Hacking's *human kinds*, "kinds are modified, revised classifications are formed, and the classified change again, loop upon loop" (Hacking, 1995, p. 370); the classifications of subjects of old age affect how individuals think of

74 *A critical enquiry into old age*

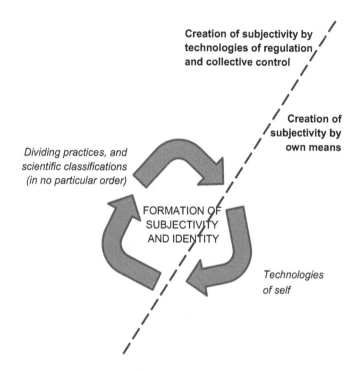

Figure 3.2 A subjectivity formation model created by merging modes of objectification (Foucault, 1982) with Hacking's looping effects (Hacking, 1995, 1999) (own illustration, 2018).

themselves, their self-worth, and how they remember their past. If we consider scientific classifications, dividing practices, and technologies of self to be three parts of the same circulatory loop of subjectivity formation, my interest lies on the side of the loop that depicts 'technologies of regulation and collective control' (Powell and Biggs, 2000), that is, how governments and disciplines study, classify, divide, and regulate individuals and groups.

I have described various national policies and projects led by the government and private sector that have been centred around the NHS, social care services, and telecare technologies. Now, I will reflect on thematising government's white papers, guidance documents, and industry reports. These publications have been referenced throughout previous sections that presented the history of telecare and social care services. The objective in this section is to find a cluster of topics that signify certain trends and reveal key themes. The key documents that have been selected are representative in: (a) reflecting rationales and preconceptions and (b) preparing the foundation for the introduction of new debates, actions, and policy changes regarding social care and care technologies.

Forewords in government and industry publications

In his book *Critical Discourse Analysis: The Critical Study of Language*, Fairclough (2010) analyses political texts, including the forewords of government documents. His aim is to "discuss theoretical perspectives on the character of contemporary politics and the State especially in advanced capitalist countries like Britain" in order to be able to analyse "dialectical relations between semiosis and other elements, especially at the level of social practices and orders of discourse" (Fairclough, 2010, p. 239). It is important to note that the forewords of the following government and industry publications (which will be thematised) offer condensed versions of the information given in the documents. These are the documents that have been used as references in the previous sections to elaborate on the history of NHS and telecare services in England.

The foreword texts in the documents have been written in a personal voice – almost speech-like – by actors such as by prime ministers or members of parliament. The use of the words 'we', 'us', and 'our' seems to be a common occurrence. In this way, the texts encapsulate a sense of inclusivity and emotiveness. This tone can give insights into "the character of contemporary politics" as described by Fairclough (2010, p. 239). Also, the inclusive use of language in the forewords align with the Foucauldian definitions of power, which depict the shift from sovereign power to disciplinary power and bio-power that generates control mechanisms over the social body.

To start the thematisation with a specific telecare document, I can give the example of the 2005 guidance paper *Building Telecare in England* (Department of Health, 2005b). This government document focusses explicitly on telecare services. It starts with a statement from the Parliamentary Under-Secretary of State for Care Services. The statement first focusses on the demographic changes that future years will bring and acknowledges that public services will face problems. In addition to statistical estimates, predictions are made about the future older population's expectations of public services. Because this information creates a sense of urgency in dealing with a somehow alarming view of the future, a suggestion is put forward to offer a viable solution that is supported by a set of justifications. Finally, supporting statements about telecare strategies are presented, as well as discussions of the uncertainty around future possibilities.

76 *A critical enquiry into old age*

A similar methodical flow of statements and similar themes can be found in several more of the government's publications on social care. In order to demonstrate similarities between documents with an attention on recurring themes, various quotations will be taken from the foreword of the *Building Telecare in England* document (Department of Health, 2005b), as well as from those forewords written by prime ministers, ministers, and secretaries of state in six other documents. These documents have been selected as a representative case from the document 'pool', which contains 40 documents.[13]

In addition to the *Building Telecare in England* paper, five of these documents have been published by the Department of Health, or by Her Majesty's Government. A brief description of these publications: (1) the 2001 strategic framework document *Quality and choice for older people's housing* (Department of Health and DETR, 2001b); (2) the 2005 green paper *Independence, Well-being and Choice* (Department of Health, 2005c); (3) the 2006 white paper *Our health, our care, our say* (Department of Health, 2006); (4) the 2009 green paper *Shaping the Future of Care Together* (HM Government, 2009); and (5) the 2010 white paper *Building the National Care Service* (HM Government, 2010). Each government paper foreword gives a glimpse of the rest of the document; a person in authority explains both the issue at hand and the solution concisely. Although these five documents do not explicitly focus on telecare, all of them encompass care and telecare technologies as part of their strategies. At the same time, each recognises older people as the primary users of social care services, and therefore the primary users of care technologies.

Similarly, the 2016 white paper, *Putting People First*, which was written by the industry body TSA (TSA, 2016a), reflects the themes discussed as part of the TSA's Think Tank Panel.[14] This panel includes third sector leads, industry consultants, and NHS and government officials – such as the Minister of State for Care Services, who acted as TSA's senior advisor. The two forewords written in this document – one by a consultant and the other by a minister – have parallels with the government's own publications, but with a stronger explicit focus on the future of care technologies observed. The forewords in this document will also be included in the thematisation process.

The previous sections in this chapter have dealt with the history of telecare, social services, and of the NHS. I presented a short overview of the seven documents in those sections, along with other policies; and now, I will refer to their forewords in this section. While laying out the quotations from the representative documents, some themes, concepts, and meanings recurred multiple times. In the first round of categorisation, each quote has been labelled with codes, then these

A critical enquiry into old age 77

codes have been turned into sub-themes. In the second round, the sub-themes have been grouped together to reflect more general trends, through which the main theme itself has been created. These main themes are as follows:

1   Categorisations of Old Age
2   Modernisation
3   Legitimising Technologies and Institutions
4   Togetherness and Social Responsibilities

The categorisation process I undertake is informed by the historical accounts and the analytical tools presented in Chapter 2. This is in line with Bryman's (2012) elaboration on theory-neutrality:

> Nowadays it is rarely accepted that theory-neutral observation is feasible. In other words, it is generally agreed that what we 'see' when we conduct research is conditioned by many factors, one of which is what we already know about the social world being studied (both in terms of social scientific conceptualizations and as members of society)
>
> (p. 574)

A list of quotes extracted from the forewords is given below, subsumed under the four primary themes. At the end of each quote is a code given in [ ] brackets and a document reference. These codes provided the grounds for creating those sub-categories that have been listed underneath the primary theme (in the form a, b, and so on).

1   Categorisations of Old Age

    a   Recognition of social issues linked with an ageing population
    b   Normalised expectations of older people
    c   Quantification of older people as a group
    d   Use of standardised measures: for example, QoL

The main theme and its secondary themes have been created based on the quotes and codes below:

I   Over the coming years, many over-65s in England will be better off and better educated, with higher expectations of public services than retirees before them. They will have been accustomed to and will expect higher quality services. (Department of Health, 2005b, p. 3)
[normalised expectations]

II They want independence, and after a life-time's work, they want, and are entitled to, dignity for life. (Department of Health, 2005b, p. 3)
[normalised expectations]

III Over the next fifty years the number of people over 65 will rise from 9.3 million to 16.8 million. (Department of Health, 2005b, p. 3)
[use of statistical/numerical data]

IV An estimated 90% of older people want to live in their own home. (Department of Health, 2005b, p. 4)
[use of statistical/numerical data]

V Research funded by the Department of Health suggests that as many as 35% of those people could be supported to live at home or in extra care housing schemes through the use of telecare. (Department of Health, 2005b, p. 4)
[use of statistical/numerical data]

VI [...] surveys suggest that the majority of people would prefer to be supported to die in their own homes. (Department of Health, 2005b, p. 4)
[use of statistical/numerical data]

VII And, of course, people do not always want to be entirely dependent on friends and family. It is in these situations that organised social care should provide the services needed to ensure wellbeing and support the independence of individuals. (Department of Health, 2005c, p. 5)
[independence]

VIII Our policies to improve housing quality and choice and modernise public services are as relevant to improving the quality of life of older people as they are for others in society. (Department of Health and DETR, 2001b, p. 4)
[quality of life]

IX We know that it will not be able to cope with future pressures in its current form and we need to reform the funding system. (HM Government, 2009, p. 4)
[recognising issues]

X The current care and support system is no longer sufficient. (HM Government, 2010, p. 2)
[recognising issues]

A critical enquiry into old age 79

XI In the depths of the Second World War, William Beveridge inspired this country to battle the five 'giant evils' of want, disease, ignorance, squalor and idleness. Today, a fear of old age is just as great a challenge. (HM Government, 2010, p. 4)
[metaphor, recognising issues]

XII People are healthier and living for longer. This is a great victory but the implication is that more people will need care and support. Left unchanged, this would push our current system of social care to breaking point. (HM Government, 2010, p. 4)
[recognising issues]

XIII We must continue adapting this support to ensure it meets people's expectations of a high-quality service and their aspirations for independence. (Department of Health, 2005c, p. 3)
[normalised expectations, independence]

XIV We face a challenge no other generation has had to confront: an ageing population rightfully demanding greater dignity, self-respect and support in old age and increasing numbers of people with disability, rightly demanding care and support which enables them to learn, work and contribute to society. (HM Government, 2010, p. 2)
[normalised expectations]

XV The current social care system was designed for a different era and cannot cope with the challenges of today. A boy born in 1951 could expect to live for 77 years, while a boy born in 2008 can expect to live until he is nearly 89. Over the next 20 years, an additional 1.7 million people in England will have a care and support need. (HM Government, 2010, p. 4)
[use of statistical/numerical data]

XVI Technology is the enabler and connector, the object is the quality of life of the patient, service user and carer." (TSA, 2016a, p. 5)
[quality of life]

2   Modernisation

   a. Reforming services
   b. Promoting independence and person-centricity[15]
   c. Choice and consumerism
   d. Privatisation

The main theme and its secondary themes have been created based on the quotes and codes below:

I   'Older people' are no different to 'younger people' in wanting choice over where and how they live their lives, and access to good quality, responsive services to enable them to live life to the full. (Department of Health and DETR, 2001b, p. 4)

[choice, service reform]

II   Our policies to improve housing quality and choice and modernise public services are as relevant to improving the quality of life of older people as they are for others in society. (Department of Health and DETR, 2001b, p. 4)

[service reform]

III   There is a rich diversity amongst our older population and a 'one size fits all' approach is no longer valid. Our aim is to set out a vision and put in place actions that will continue the process of innovation and development so that older people are offered higher quality and more choice over their housing and services wherever they live. (Department of Health and DETR, 2001b, p. 4)

[service reform, choice]

IV   In this endeavour we are working closely with a wide range of organisations in the statutory, voluntary and private sectors. There is much activity outside Government that is seeking appropriate solutions, and we want to harness and co-ordinate this work with our own. We can achieve far more for older people through a partnership approach than we could alone. (Department of Health and DETR, 2001b, p. 4)

[partnership with private sector, justification]

V   This is an important part of our commitment to renew and modernise all our public services so they are centred on the needs and wishes of the individual. (Department of Health, 2005c, p. 3)

[service reform]

VI   Our society, quite rightly, values the independence that we all try to develop as adults: our own income, our own family and our own choices for leisure, meals and lifestyle. (Department of Health, 2005c, p. 6)

[independence, choice, consumerism]

VII   People will be helped in their goal to remain healthy and independent. (Department of Health, 2006, p. 4)

[independence]

VIII   That is why GPs are being given greater control over their budgets and will be more accountable for the money they spend. This will allow them to acquire for their patients services from a broader range of providers within the NHS, voluntary and private sector. (Department of Health, 2006, p. 1)
[partnership with private sector]

IX   Services will be integrated, built round the needs of individuals and not service providers, promoting independence and choice. (Department of Health, 2006, p. 4)
[independence, choice]

X   People will have real choices and greater access in both health and social care. (Department of Health, 2006, p. 4)
[choice]

XI   The current care and support system was designed in the 1940s and we need to develop a system that fits our needs in the 21st century. We need a system that is fairer, simpler and more affordable for everyone. (HM Government, 2009, p. 4)
[service reform]

XII   [About the Big Care Debate] People told us that the time for reform has come. They told us they need a system that will support them and their families to live the lives they want, that will treat everyone with dignity and respect and that will give them choice and control over their care. (HM Government, 2010, p. 4)
[working together, public consultation, choice and control]

XIII   This White Paper is not about technology: it is about people. (TSA, 2016a, p. 5)
[person-centricity]

XIV   We all have a clear opportunity to embed technology within every element of care and support, and instil a 'think technology first' culture throughout our collective workforce. (TSA, 2016a, p. 4)
[service reform]

XV   Instead of focusing on technology, focus on meeting the needs of the patient, service user and carer. (TSA, 2016a, p. 5)
[person-centricity]

3   Legitimising Technologies and Institutions

    a   Recognising challenges
    b   Reassurance about future success with technologies

c Building confidence in national and local bodies
d Emphasis on localism

The main theme and its secondary themes have been created based on the quotes and codes below:

I Local authorities have a key role to play here in taking the lead locally. (Department of Health and DETR, 2001b, p. 4)
[localism]

II Telecare is vital to unlocking this future. (Department of Health, 2005b, p. 3)
[suggesting a solution]

III Throughout the consultation, the need to find a balance between the use of technology and the continuation of human contact has been a recurring theme. (Department of Health, 2005b, p. 5)
[recognising challenges/uncertainty]

IV We must take care not to allow these new technologies to control or isolate us and whilst the world around us is fast changing our basic human needs remain the same. Some care services will always be, quite rightly, delivered personally. (Department of Health, 2005b, p. 5)
[recognising challenges/uncertainty]

V None of this will be easy. Nor was slashing waiting lists, but the NHS has risen magnificently to this challenge. (Department of Health, 2006, p. 2)
[recognising challenges/uncertainty, reassurance]

VI It is a tough challenge. But we have already seen in social care how the use of direct payments, for example, has helped improve services and transform lives. (Department of Health, 2005c, p. 3)
[recognising challenges, reassurance]

VII There are innovative 'pilot projects' where we can catch a glimpse of the future and many of these have informed our vision. (Department of Health, 2005c, p. 7)
[reassurance]

VIII Previous governments have aspired to parts of this vision. But we are the first government to lay out both a comprehensive and compelling vision of preventative and empowering health and social care services and an effective programme for making this vision a reality. (Department of Health, 2006, p. 4)
[reassurance]

A critical enquiry into old age 83

IX   We will cut back the bureaucracy so local government and the NHS work effectively in tandem, and give customers a bigger voice over the care they receive. (Department of Health, 2006, p. 2)

[localism]

X   Our answer is bold, ambitious reform to create a system rooted firmly in the proudest traditions of our National Health Service. Its creation in 1948 wasn't just one of Britain's proudest moments; it was also a profound statement of what can be achieved through collective will in the face of adversity. (HM Government, 2010, p. 2)

[suggesting a solution, reassurance]

XI   This White Paper truly represents the beginnings of a profound change. (Department of Health, 2006, p. 4)

[reassurance]

XII But we will go further. (HM Government, 2010, p. 5)

[reassurance]

XIII This is an historic reform, bold and far-reaching. (HM Government, 2010, p. 5)

[reassurance]

XIV Together, we have shaped the future of care. Now is the time to take action. (HM Government, 2010, p. 5)

[reassurance]

XV   Local government's strength comes from its closeness to the communities it serves. The National Care Service will bind this with a new vision of more personalised care for everyone, focused on keeping people well and independent. (HM Government, 2010, p. 5)

[localism]

XVI I have witnessed first-hand how [technology enabled care services] can play a key part in maintaining independence and instilling confidence in family members wanting to remain in their own home and community. (TSA, 2016a, p. 4)

[reassurance]

XVII The TSA has identified a need to set up a local digital leaders' network (...) [and] will draw together local expertise and national system leaders to spread the expertise and help shape future procurement and contracting. (TSA, 2016a, p. 5)

[suggesting a solution, localism]

84 *A critical enquiry into old age*

  4 Togetherness and Social Responsibilities
      a Emphasis on intergenerational links
      b Identifying threat factors upon which the provision of care depends
      c Emphasis on moral and ethics of caring for old age

The main theme and its secondary themes have been created based on the quotes and codes below:

I   It is family and friends, of course, who still take on most of the caring responsibilities. This support is given willingly but must not be taken for granted. (Department of Health, 2005c, p. 3)
                  [threat factor]

II   We all know the challenges to which public services will have to rise. People are living longer but are less likely to have the support of an extended family. (Department of Health, 2005b, p. 3)
                  [threat factor]

III   The nation depends upon the emotions and care that we all give to the people we know. If this relationship were to disappear, organised social care could not cope. We must never forget that. (Department of Health, 2005c, p. 6)
                  [intergenerational links, threat factor]

IV   By giving frontline professionals and the public more say and control over the services they provide and receive, I am confident that we will continue building a high-quality health and social care system. (Department of Health, 2006, p. 2)
                  [working together]

V   People told us that everyone in society shares the responsibility for making sure that people receive the care they need. (HM Government, 2009, p. 4)
                  [intergenerational links, working together]

VI   These changes will affect any care that you and your family receive, so we want to know what you think. We invite you to join the Big Care Debate.16 Let's shape the future of care together. (HM Government, 2009, p. 5)
                  [working together]

VII   To build this, we will need to make some big decisions and reach agreement across society on the right way forward for England. So, this is the beginning of a Big Care Debate. (HM Government, 2009, p. 4)
                  [working together]

VIII The enormous sacrifices of the wartime generation demanded that there had to be an ambitious programme for quality healthcare, alongside economic reconstruction. Now that same generation is owed a further debt of dignity: to receive care and to stay in their homes as long as possible. (HM Government, 2010, p. 2)
[intergenerational links, morals and ethics]

IX Caring for older people and those who need support is the hallmark of civilised society." (HM Government, 2010, p. 2)
[morals and ethics]

X It is not right that people already struggling with the loss of independence – who have worked hard all their lives and saved for their retirement – are forced to run down their savings or sell their homes to fund their care. So this is a new chapter in the story of our welfare state: a chance to change the way care and support are delivered. (HM Government, 2010, p. 3)
[morals and ethics]

XI To ensure that the National Care Service can provide high quality care, free when people need it, for generations to come, the Government believes it is right that everyone should contribute. (HM Government, 2010, p. 4)
[intergenerational links, working together]

The following table summarises the primary themes and subcategories as identified in the forewords. These themes reflect the most commonly occurring topics in the representative publications, in explicitly or implicitly stated ways. Many of the themes identified reflect parallels with the review of Chapter 2, such as the problematisations of ageing, a move towards a person-centred system in health and social care, and the intergenerational social contract between generations.

The illustrations and case descriptions inside the documents

In this section, themes will be drawn from the messages in government publications that are conveyed through the use of illustrations, diagrams, case descriptions, and quote bubbles. The analysis of illustrations and visualised forms of texts are important because they reveal new meanings that may not have been directly or explicitly stated in text. For example, even though Fairclough's focus in his critical discourse analysis approach is directed upon the verbal elements of communication, he reflects that, "very often visuals and 'verbals' operate in a mutually reinforcing way which makes them very difficult to disentangle" (Fairclough, 1989, p. 28). It is common in discourse

86 *A critical enquiry into old age*

Table 3.1 List of themes: forewords

Main themes	Sub-themes
Categorisations of old age	Recognition of social issues linked with an ageing population
	Normalised expectations of older people
	Quantification of older people as a group
	Use of standardised measures e.g. QoL
Modernisation	Reforming services
	Promoting independence and person-centricity
	Choice and consumerism
	Privatisation
Legitimising technologies and institutions	Recognising challenges
	Reassurance about future success with technologies
	Building confidence in national and local bodies
	Emphasis on localism
Togetherness and social responsibilities	Emphasis on intergenerational links
	Identifying threat factors upon which the provision of care depends
	Emphasis on morals and ethics of caring for old age

analysis to examine aspects of culture as expressed through media, both as support for text and on their own (Giaschi, 2000).

The visual materials grouped in this section[17] have been detached from white papers, green papers, guidance documents, flyers, and easy-read government documents.[18] The specific visual elements have been extracted from the documents based on their capacity to convey implicit or explicit messages that relate primarily to telecare technologies, as well as to the discussions about older people. Moreover, the themes identified in the foreword analysis have given cues as to what general topics are expressed in these publications.

Overall, 25 diagrams, illustrations, case descriptions, and other visual materials have been analysed. 'Person-centric care', 'feeling in control of own care', 'independence', 'choice', and 'prevention' are the key words that have appeared the most frequently.

In this section, the illustrations, diagrams, case descriptions, and quote bubbles have been clustered into themes. It is important to note that the four themes which emerged in the foreword textual analysis recurred in the visual representations as well – with similar, yet distinct, sub-categories, as identified in the table above. In addition to the four themes, two additional categories have emerged in this section.

Because the focus on absences or omissions has been an ongoing process during document analysis, an absent theme has been noted in the analysis of visual elements. None of the visual elements in the

Table 3.2 List of themes: visual representations

Main themes	Sub-themes	Code of the visual exhibits (as given in the Appendices)
Categorisations of old age	Classification by dependence/independence	B.1, B.8, B.9
	Older people as a burden	B.7
	Older people as vulnerable	B.15
	Classification of older people versus working-age people	B.7
	Quantification of older people as a financially secure group	B.7
Modernisation	Choice, control, self-care	B.5, B.8, B.25
	Independence and person-centricity	B.4, B.6, B.8, B.23
Legitimising technologies and institutions	Building confidence in technologies through case studies	B.9, B.10, B.11, B.12, B.17, B.19, B.22
	Introducing telecare technologies through descriptions	B.13, B.14, B.15, B.16
	Gatekeeping services through new roles given to professionals	B.13, B.15
	Financial justifications	B.13, B.23
Togetherness and social responsibilities	Togetherness	B.2
	Intergenerational links	B.7
Public accounts of technology experiences	First-hand accounts of positive experiences with telecare services	B.3, B.6, B.18, B.19, B.20, B.24
	Second-hand accounts of positive experiences with telecare services	B.9, B.11, B.12, B.17
	Accounts of adverse experiences with telecare services [Absent Theme]	N/A
Care management	Risk assessments	B.13, B.14
	Financial evaluations of services	B.13, B.23, B.25

selected 40 documents have addressed the accounts of adverse experiences with telecare, neither as a first-hand or second-hand account from older people who have been using care technologies. This leads to a noticeable partiality, because the visual accounts of positive experiences have been overwhelmingly deployed in the publications.

Summary

To sum up, the following themes have emerged out of the analysis of governmental care policies:

1 Categorisations of old age
2 Modernisation
3 Legitimising technologies and institutions
4 Togetherness and social responsibilities
5 Public accounts of technology experiences
6 Care management

Regrouping these themes in terms of their relation to the questions can be helpful. Two overarching themes are observed within the data that have been divided into six main themes; they can be collected under: *(1) Classifications, practices, and processes*, and *(2) Identity*. With the use of such a model, the processes of *dividing practices* and *scientific classifications* can be identified under the first theme; and how these processes reflect on *old age identities* can be identified under the second.

However, there is a third and final overarching theme – *(3) Social responsibilities* – which also emerged out of the data in a compelling way. This theme is linked to the first two themes and has the potential to lead to an interesting analysis. Figure 3.3 visually presents the relationships between the main themes and those overarching themes that have been generated based on the need for more clarification towards the three guiding questions. They were refined as follows:

Q1: Through which scientific classification practices do old age discourses surface in relation to telecare?
Q2: Through which dividing practices do old age discourses surface in relation to telecare?
Q3: How do social care policies enact and transform the grand narratives and the identity of old age?

The descriptive aspects of the six main themes, as well as the identification of scientific classifications and dividing practices, mainly fall under the first overarching theme, *Classifications, practices, and processes*. The main discussion of the discursive aspects of these themes falls under the second overarching theme, *Old age identity*. The third overarching theme, *Social responsibilities*, draws from the main theme of the same name. It has a significant place because of the distinct ways in which this theme has appeared in data. Investigating any overlapping or contradictory trends present in the relationship between *Classifications, practices, and processes* and *Social responsibilities* will

A critical enquiry into old age 89

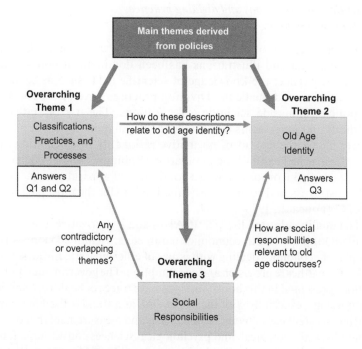

Figure 3.3 Dividing the aspects of primary themes into further overarching themes (Own illustration, 2019).

play a part in the next sections. My aim is to connect the three overarching themes together in a meaningful and sequential manner.

Classifications, practices, and processes

In the previous section, the analysis and categorisation of data revealed that older people are identified as a distinct demographic group. This distinction is observable in the various policies and strategies that aimed to create changes or introduce new technologies for old age assistance or old age care. There are indications that old age is constructed as a distinct kind. I will elaborate on the techniques (modes) through which the dominant discourses of old age have surfaced. The second objective is to reflect upon the construction of this distinct identity and human kind (Hacking, 1995, 1999). This second task also includes the recognition of changes in the historical grand discourses of old age and in relation to the discourses of old age that have formed in the context of telecare technologies.

Scientific classifications and dividing practices embedded in policies

The quantification of older people through the use of numerical and statistical data and illustrations has been dominant in policies that collectively reflect the knowledge of scientific fields such as economics, statistics, and medicine. Dividing practices have also been used in policies alongside scientific classifications. The use of statistical methods and judgements that divide the population in the era of biopower shows the spread of normative rationality in calculating and monitoring the health of the population (Rabinow, 1984). Policies are "increasingly incorporated into a continuum of apparatuses (medical, administrative, and so on) whose functions are for the most part regulatory" (Foucault, 1980a, p. 144).

The quality adjusted life year (QALY) and its derivative, the quality of life (QoL), are health economics parameters. Health economics is a branch of economics dealing with issues of efficiency, effectiveness, and value in healthcare provision and consumption. The governmental publications presented in this book's analysis have traces of health economics terminology, especially with the use of *QoL* as a standardised measure. Their consistent use of methods of analysis and measurement that derive from physical, biological, and psychological sciences constitutes a form of scientific classification. While the term 'quality of life' can apply to a range of things (each reflecting different perspectives), its application as something that can be measured through methods of quantification is an economics approach, which contains embedded hierarchies of value as to what constitutes 'quality' in the eyes of the measurer. Statistics, in particular, are a form of data used heavily and frequently in these documents. For example, future projections (e.g. population growth forecasts) depend on official statistics, which originate from the UK's largest independent producer of statistics, The Office for National Statistics. Moreover, as an example of deployed techniques that render qualitative information into quantifiable data, surveys have been identified as the most frequently used method of data collection from older people. In such cases of scientific classification, the use of statistical information and quantifying tools within the policies also make visible the financial aspects of old age discourses.

Financial justifications and financial data are also used to support the case for telecare. This is another technique of scientific classification that sets up a dichotomy of 'cost effective' versus 'costly' forms of care and then views or problematises old age through these terms. However, this classification technique has only been sparsely used in policies, as evidenced in the case study. This could be linked to the fact that no compelling results were presented by the scientific studies regarding the large-scale telecare trial, Whole System Demonstrator (WSD), during the period when telecare became more visible. These studies conducted economic evaluations of the WSD's telecare service with the use of randomised control trials, and reflected that no significant outcomes were observed (Steventon et al., 2013; Henderson et al., 2014). The infrequent occurrence of cost-effectiveness of telecare as a measure in the case study reinforces the view that cost-effectiveness data are especially limited in the UK (Henderson et al., 2014).

However, in the absence of wider financial justifications about the use of telecare by older people, there has been a strong focus on highlighting the positive experiences that older people have with telecare services. This technique of reporting on positive telecare experiences can be classified as a dividing practice of standardisation and normalisation. That is because this selective highlighting of positive cases and findings categorises *care with telecare* as the 'standard', 'normal', and favourable experience for the older population. Since the economic evaluations of telecare are used sparingly due to their ambivalent results, the case of telecare has been supported on governmental documents with qualitative data such as answers given to questionnaires or public accounts collected through think tanks.

Case studies have been dominantly used in policy papers. They reflect an objective to build confidence in telecare technologies through the use of narratives, such as self-management, independence, risk management (such as reducing the risk of being referred to intensive care), falls prevention, the prevention of delayed discharges, and the protection of the most vulnerable. The use of such narratives reflects another objectification practice that divides the older people (a) from the rest of the population and (b) from each other, as distinct sub-groups (e.g. identification as 'able-bodied' or 'disabled'; as 'independent' or 'dependent', and so on) within the 'older population' category. This practice creates institutionalised objects with particular attributes in relation to telecare.

Adverse experiences with telecare technologies have not been accounted for in policy and strategy documents. There have been academic discussions in sociology and bioethics about the surveillance aspects of telecare technologies, as well as the compliance logics that are embedded in these technologies (Schermer, 2009; Guta et al., 2012; Sorell and Draper, 2012). It has been observed that no critique has been used in policy that may lead to negative or ambivalent meanings about telecare.

An absence of discussions has been spotted about topics, such as why traditional care still matters; how telecare could change certain aspects of society, such as monitoring and surveillance; and how to overcome the potentially coercive effects that telecare could create (e.g. an increase in family neglect/isolation for older relatives due to confidence in technologies). In addition to a marked absence of these themes, certain scientific approaches – such as the classifications of the sociology field – have been left at the margins of the dominant narratives upon which these policies were constructed. The dominant assertions were based predominantly on economic, statistical, and medical knowledge.

Although metaphors are uncommon in the policies, one specific metaphor found in the foreword of a governmental white paper creates a powerful narrative about attitudes towards ageing:

> In the depths of the Second World War, William Beveridge inspired this country to battle the five 'giant evils' of want, disease, ignorance, squalor and idleness. Today, a fear of old age is just as great a challenge.
>
> (HM Government, 2010, p. 4)

Here, the fear of old age is problematised and is classified as a 'giant evil' that should be battled – as something undesired and to be wished away. In Katz's words, problematisations signify "the disciplinary practices that transform a realm of human existence into a crisis of thought" (1996, p. 9). It has been observed that dividing practices are typically supported by disciplinary and scientific classifications to normalise the separations.

For example, other powerful themes that I discovered in my critical enquiry were the visions of: (1) older people as a burden, (2) older versus working-age people, and (3) older people as a financially secure group. These three narratives have been deployed to support each other. The statistical categorisation of "those aged between 65 and 74 [as] the second wealthiest age group in Britain" (HM Government, 2010, p. 128), with the use of data from the Office for National Statistics, indicates a scientific classification practice that uses the knowledge of a centralised statistics authority. With this classification, the aim is to support the two dividing practices that have been used in the same context: those that (1) position older people against working-age people and (2) divide them from society as a burden on the shoulders of younger people. By implication, referring to younger people as *working-age people* reduces older people to an unproductive/passive population. Hence the narrative of being a burden becomes inextricably linked with the *work* narrative.

To justify the financially secure position of older people, the same extract states that "by contrast, many younger people have significant debts from mortgages or student loans" (HM Government, 2010,

p. 128). This statement creates a theoretical division in population in terms of wealth accumulation. Furthermore, as a result of reductionism and homogenisation of the population, only two primary categories are put forward by policies: younger vs older people. Because the division is reductive, this distinction filters out the heterogeneous realities of social life. First, the data from the Office for National Statistics state that wealth is highest amongst the age group 45–65, which surpasses the age group 65–74 (ONS, 2013). Since the governmental definitions of old age concerns those individuals 65 and over, the most financially secure age group in Britain (45–64) are, in principle, part of the 'younger' population, thereby also under the 'burden' of supporting the older generations. This creates a contradiction with the financially insecure image of younger people, through which an element of 'unfairness' between generations has been introduced into the policies.

Second, on the back of the *care caps* and *means tests*, the conditions of how older people are supported can be unpredictable. Echoing Loopstra et al.'s study (2016), the cuts in welfare spending and changes in care caps and means tests can lead to precarious conditions for older people. This implies that the wealth of the 65+ age group is in a precarious position in relation to changing laws. One example is the decreasing number of people who are receiving publicly funded social care from 2010 onwards (Fernandez et al., 2013; King's Fund and Nuffield Trust, 2016); this is not a result of people having higher wealth accumulation, but due to people being deemed as ineligible to receive funds under the changing rules.

Third, statements that explicitly or implicitly separate the younger and older population, and categorise older people as a burden contradict other narratives: for example, those that convey a youthful image of older people and blur the boundaries of age differences. This can be seen in quotes such as "Older people are no different to younger people in wanting choice over where and how they live their lives" (Department of Health and DETR, 2001b, p. 4). The 'old age as a burden' discourse is also in contradiction with the narratives of morality and social responsibilities between generations, which emerge out of the same policies and strategies.

Modernisation of services

The modernisation and reformation of social care services has been a dominant theme in the majority of policies. This reflects a cluster of structural processes and relations in social care that relate to old age and telecare. As part of the descriptions of modernisation in policies, certain narratives have emerged, which include themes such as promoting independence, person-centricity, choice, and control.

The modernisation of services narrative echoes the logics of privatisation. It has been explicitly stated in policies that governments have been working closely with other sectors, including the voluntary and private sector. A governmental foreword reflects that "There is much activity outside Government that is seeking appropriate solutions, and we want to harness and co-ordinate this work with our own. We can achieve far more for older people through a partnership approach than we could alone" (Department of Health and DETR, 2001b, p. 4). As discussed in the history of health and social care services in England, there is a link between efforts to modernise (in particular, to finance modernisation) in recent decades and an increasing entanglement with private finance initiatives (PFIs). I will now elaborate on how the attempts to define modernisation in those policies regarding old age and telecare highlight the shift towards a specific form of government, which has been defined by Estes and Linkins (1997) as the 'hollow state'.

As identified earlier, 'hollow state' refers to the separation between the central government and the services that the government funds. In this model, the central government contracts out the provision of services to other bodies and keeps for itself the monitoring and inspection responsibilities. The policies reflect a certain form of hollow state formation because the social care responsibilities are being shifted towards the local level authorities, namely the councils; and commissioning happens at these local levels. National policies guide some aspects of service provision; however, the local authorities can enact the policies in a variety of ways, including forming partnerships with different private organisations.

An example of an external body that works alongside the telecare providing social care services is the Telecare Services Association (TSA) – the only telecare accreditation body in England. This not-for-profit community interest company is responsible for establishing quality standards for telecare services in England, and they have been gaining more momentum after having been publicly endorsed by the government. TSA has substantial sway and no viable competitors in their role, and this indicates a monopoly that corresponds to the notion of the hollow state. These findings align with the post-Thatcher era changes advocated in the UK by successive governments that shifted long-term care for older people from the NHS onto the local authorities (Scott-Samuel et al., 2014). This shows that localism has been given a special emphasis in policies; one of the key presuppositions of hollow state is the reliance of the state on local bodies.

It has been observed that *technological care* has been presented under the theme of *modernisation* in the policies, thus implicitly associating the elements of independence, person-centricity, choice, and control with the technologies. The analysis in this book aligns with Klecun's observation about the technology discourse being intertwined with the discourse of patient-centred care and person-centricity, which at first appears implicitly in earlier publications, and then explicitly in later publications (Klecun, 2016). This was the case with the government's publications from 2010 onwards, in which such language around technologies has been more overt, signifying a more dominant narrative of technologies in social care.

Independence is a common recurring topic that has been taken up in all policies relating to technologies. The quote that refers to the government's definition of independence in the most explicit way is: "Our society, quite rightly, values the independence that we all try to develop as adults: our own income, our own family and our own choices for leisure, meals and lifestyle" (Department of Health, 2005c, p. 6). Resourcefulness through own income, own family, and own choices for services and lifestyles thus become the elements upon which the independence is constructed. By implication, dependency refers to those situations where the older individuals use other resources for their care than their own income; rely largely on state's social care services rather than on their own family; and are not on the lookout for the most prudent services and lifestyles. The policies also state that "people will be helped in their goal to remain healthy and independent" (Department of Health, 2006, p. 4), where the use of the phrase 'their goal' infers a method to create implicit compliance, through which the above definition of independence is normalised and standardised in the population.

The government pronounces their commitment to "modernise all [their] public services so they are centred on the needs and wishes of the individual" (Department of Health, 2005c, p. 3); person-centricity and personalisation are the themes reflected here. As studied by Wakefield and Fleming (2009), the narrative of personalisation has been widening in the late modernity to include such catchwords as *personal choice* and *control*. The aim is to empower individuals and render them responsible for certain tasks, which have been previously recognised as a responsibility of other bodies or have not been recognised as a responsibility at all. This type of 'responsibilisation' (Wakefield and Fleming, 2009; Lim, 2012) is heavily implied in the policies because the subsequent governments have transferred responsibilities to individuals and families, who are then expected to take an active role in resolving their own problems.

To illustrate: choosing from the range of adult social care services offered in an individual's local authority is the responsibility of the individual. Social care services have not been free at the point of delivery in England. Local authority support is means-tested, and the individuals who receive funding are expected to contribute towards the cost of their care (Jarrett, 2017). Since older people are the primary users of the social care services,[19] their responsibility over their own care reflects that the responsibilisation process of the social care in England primarily targets the older population. The aforementioned phrase 'their goal' (Department of Health, 2006, p. 4) also reflects an instance of responsibilisation. This echoes Phillipson's statement about how the understanding of ageing is associated with "how individuals rather than societies handle the demands associated with social ageing" (Phillipson, 1998, p. 119).

I have previously stated that, with the hollow state model, the government contracts out the provision of services to other bodies but keeps the monitoring responsibilities. Parallels can be drawn between these theorisations of the hollow state and responsibilisation. The definition of the hollow state notes that the duties of government are outsourced to other institutions, and responsibilisation describes self-responsibility (a person's responsibility over their own care). It can be concluded that responsibilisation is intricately linked with the logic of the hollow state, because, by implication, the care duties of the welfare state are contracted out from the central government to the local councils and on to the individuals themselves.

Care management

The arrival of managerialism in the UK social welfare system in the 1990s marked a shift in social welfare in which "central control has been replaced by local power; management systems are inspired by consumer and market models; there is a reliance on risk assessment; and an increase in the discourses of a 'politics of participation' and 'social inclusion'" (Powell and Biggs, 2000, p. 4). Various instances of care managerialism manifested in policies during my analysis.

Managerialism primarily relies on risk assessments, and this is done at the local authority level in the domain of adult social care services. Before the installation of telecare in individual homes, assessments take place in the houses to investigate and classify the conditions of people, and match these 'cases' with appropriate solutions. Older people are also financially assessed to access telecare services, based on *care caps* and *means tests*, whose configurations remain uncertain given the possible policy changes. When individuals are considered as 'cases' in these ways, they are "described, judged, measured, compared with others" so that they can "be trained, classified, normalised, excluded" (Foucault, 1977, p. 191).

As Powell and Biggs state "central control has been replaced by local power; management systems are inspired by consumer and market models; there is a reliance on risk assessment" (2000, p. 4). Foucault argues that 'assessment', as a disciplinary technique, aims to describe, judge, measure, and compare older people with the use of norms and by "imposing new delimitations on them" (Foucault, 1977, p. 184). An assessment can be considered to be a central technique that makes an individual into an object of power/knowledge (Foucault, 1977). It can thus be argued that, through assessments, ageing bodies are constituted in relation to normalised standards of risks, and older people are rendered into objects of economic and social narratives that address 'financial resources' and required levels of 'supervision' (Powell and Biggs, 2000).

The telecare alarms and sensors present at individuals' homes are the products of the aforementioned risk assessments conducted by local authorities. Through the assessment and the implementation of technologies, more links are created between homes and telecare monitoring centres, enabling more interactions between older people and professionals, and more data collection about them. This implies that a greater level of monitoring takes place over service users, and that a higher dependency on telecare services is generated. This sort of reliance demonstrates that the narrative of 'independence' via telecare is not self-referential; it reflects specific governmental and managerial values, and is therefore limited.

The consolidation of managerialism in the management of old age creates changes in the welfare apparatuses (Warnes, 1996). As Becks (1992) states, reflexive modernity/postmodernity separates individuals from collective structures. The dissolution of boundaries of the welfare state's collective structures in the neoliberal era can shift the focus from certain elements in life onto flexibilities and 'choices'. This aligns with the reflection that neoliberalism's main function is to self-govern (Fukuyama, 1996; Rose, 1999).

The marketisation of telecare is legitimised through the narratives of 'choice' and 'independence'. The narrative that presents itself in several policies and treats service users as 'clients' can lead to the same effects of marketisation as seen in the private sector. The inclusion of BT – as a private company – in earlier telecare projects has been an indicator of an early trend. It has been demonstrated in Chapter 2 that local authorities are working more closely with private sector organisations, as in the examples of alliances formed with Telecare Choice (provider of telecare services) and Tunstall Healthcare (provider of technology).

These partnerships shape the ways telecare services are delivered, and this implies that specific designs and functionalities are being normalised and institutionalised. A potential hazard can arise for the service users if private organisations standardise their services without the complete knowledge of local demands, networks, and historical practices. Moreover, in those regions where robust telecare initiatives have not been initiated by local authorities, private organisations could become the leading providers for telecare services; and this, in turn, would make the services of local authorities redundant. The private sector is likely to operate on a different set of values and competition logics. On the one hand, there is a potential upside to this competition in that it can promote the providers to meet higher standards and better offers for older people. However, the potential downside is that it can promote them to look for more 'cost-effective' options.

Social responsibilities

The theme of social responsibilities and intergenerational links appeared in an interesting way. Even though the logics of modernisation and of care management are rationalised in alignment with the shifts in the era of a neoliberal (post)welfare state, the narrative of social responsibilities seems to have appeared in contradiction with other powerful narratives.

The white paper published after the 2009 Big Care Debate public consultation states that people from the public who joined the Big Care Debate told the government "that everyone in society shares the responsibility for making sure that people receive the care they need" (HM Government, 2009, p. 4). The paper also recognises the fact that older people "are forced to run down their savings or sell their homes to fund their care" (HM Government, 2010, p. 3), and it calls for changes in how the welfare state functions. These statements deem social care as a collective duty, and they reflect upon it as a reinforcing element of the 'intergenerational contract'.

However, indications of ambivalent attitudes have also been noted in discussions about social responsibilities in policies. For example, in the same government publications, the unfairness between generations has been highlighted in this reference to the tax-funded system: "The majority of people to benefit from a fully tax-funded system would be older people, and yet it is working-age adults who would face the largest burden in paying for it" (HM Government, 2010, p. 128). This echoes Phillipson's (1998) argument about how an increasing number of workers are disinclined to pay tax increases to support benefits for older people, and by doing so they were breaking the 'intergenerational contract'. This reflects late modernity's separation of individuals from collective structures (Becks, 1992), through which individualisation sets agency free from the social structures of simple modernity (Lash, 1994).

It has been observed that the narrative of unfairness between generations is outweighed by manifold other accounts regarding familial and societal care, as well as the ethical responsibilities of the population. The foreword analysis has revealed that governmental publications use phrases such as 'caring responsibilities', 'debt of dignity owed to wartime generation', and 'caring for older people as the hallmark of civilised society'. The publications explicitly state that the nation depends upon the emotions and care that people give to the others they know (Department of Health, 2005c), but that the support of family and friends must not be taken for granted (Department of Health, 2005c).

The phrase "enormous sacrifices of the wartime generation[20]" (HM Government, 2010, p. 2) echoes the previous discussion about productivity, as indicated within the *dividing practice* of working-age versus older people. With this, the individuals under the pension age are homogenised as the productive and active population which comprises taxpayers. With the "enormous sacrifices of the wartime generation", it is implied that then working-age people were active and productive, and now they make up the 'deserving old'. This aligns with Phillipson's argument about "harsh or softer versions of dependency" (Phillipson, 1998), such as the concept of older people as a problem population, or as deserving of a reward for their past contributions to society. A softer version of dependency is constructed here with the narrative of 'sacrifices of older generation' and 'a debt of dignity owed to them' by later generations.

Another dependency is created through statements indicating that older people should be supported to stay in their homes as long as possible, and that familial care should not be taken for granted. Since the objective of the policies is to announce the new strategies in social care services like telecare, these narratives of staying in the home and the decreasing levels of familial support feed those grounds upon which telecare is legitimised. Even though a number of national level documentations recognise telecare as a complementary form of care, as opposed to something that replaces or substitutes human contact, the discussion about what types of care that telecare is complementing has been lacking in depth.

I identified how several compelling themes and narratives that have been emphasised in policies are in accordance with the notion of an emerging 'hollow state' (Estes and Linkins, 1997). These are: (1) the late modernity's key component of social change, which is individualisation

(Becks, 1992); (2) the logics of consumerism and privatisation in social care; and (3) the responsibilisation of life that denotes self-responsibility over choices and lifestyles (Wakefield and Fleming, 2009). It has also been stated that the understanding of ageing is becoming more associated with "how individuals rather than societies handle the demands associated with social ageing" (Phillipson, 1998, p. 119). These themes appear to be in contradiction with the narrative around the intergenerational contract based on morality between the generations. The technologies are legitimised and normalised in rational ways, and the theme of togetherness and morality presents itself as a traditional narrative in various spaces of this rationality.

The narrative of social responsibility reflects a traditional discourse that is ambivalent and shifting in its position. We can turn our attention to the wider political and social context, including the reality of neoliberal modernisation and care management values. When we put social responsibilities against the narrative of individualisation and individual responsibilities – which occurred heavily in the analysis of modernisation and care management – the social responsibility discourse is shown to hold conflicting meanings.

As Foucault argues, discontinuities in discourses happen when things are no longer perceived, classified, and known in the same way as before (Foucault, 1994b). The presence of ambiguities and ambivalent positions within policy texts indicate that the narrative of social responsibility and of the intergenerational contract might be gradually dissolving, although it is evidently not a discontinuous discourse. The continuity of the social responsibility discourse still manifests itself in policies. It carries the traces of the moral framework that had been constructed in the post-war welfare state period. Foucault reflects that some of the discourse would be continuous over time, until society establishes the new form of truth based on the steady accumulation of knowledge (Foucault, 1994b). Until that time, the discourse of social responsibility and intergenerational morality will constitute an implicit vehicle, and a powerful narrative, through which the conflicting logics and processes of social care modernisation will be carried forward, while appealing to traditional community values.

Old age identity

Foucault (1982) argues that subjectification forms a process that categorises the individual, and that the individual becomes a carrier of meaning (Dagg and Haugaard, 2016). The individuality of the person is marked with this meaning, giving them a particular identity – a particular way of being. The public policies reveal explicit and implicit ways of positioning older people that bestow on them particular old age identities.

A critical enquiry into old age 101

With old age identity, I refer to an *abstraction/representation* of an old age identity. In the critical enquiry conducted in this book, this identity is constituted by those power/knowledge formations that impose a form of control structure upon old age subjects through the medium of care policies. To construct an old age identity, it is necessary to: (1) refer to the discourses, as well as the effects of certain structural processes and relations (modernisation and care management), which contribute to the particular social positioning of older people, and (2) reveal those enactments of and alterations (if any) to the grand discourses of old age on the back of the discourses and processes identified.

The following table presents the discourses, structural processes and relations pertaining to old age, which have surfaced with the scientific classifications and dividing practices previously identified.

Various discourses of old age are present in the context of telecare, which are mediated through policies and strategies. The majority of these discourses can be positioned under the grand discourses of old age because they can be deemed as sub-discourses within the grand discourse itself. To mark these similarities, I build on Figure 2.1 from Chapter 2 and position the discourses and processes from Table 3.3 as enactments of the grand discourses. To echo Foucault's statement: "there is nothing to be gained from describing this autonomous layer of

Table 3.3 List of identified discourses and processes relating to old age

Manifestations of old age discourses in policies and strategies	*Manifestations of social care and old age-related structural processes and relations*
1 Fear of old age as an 'evil' to battle	12 Old age as an economic variable
2 Old age as a burden	13 Consumerism in old age
3 Old age as the unproductive population	14 Hollow state
4 Older people as a financially secure group	15 Responsibilisation and individualisation
5 Old age dependency as the source of unfairness between generations	16 Dependency on telecare institutions and professionals
6 Old age as risk	17 Empowerment through personal choices
7 Being independent with own resources	18 Risk assessments
8 Older people as youthful	19 Staying at home as long as possible
9 The deserving old	20 Marketisation of services
10 The heroic old	21 Localism
11 Intergenerational debt	

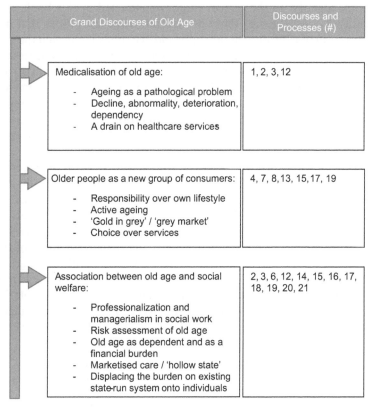

Figure 3.4 Classifying discourses, processes, and relations under the grand discourses of old age (own illustration, 2019).

discourses unless one can relate it to other layers, practices, institutions, social relations, political relations, and so on" (Foucault, 1967, p. 284 in O'Farrell, 2005). This calls for the recognition of other objects beyond discourse, although their relationship with the discourse is primary. I use the components of Table 3.3 to demonstrate those enactments of the grand discourses. Figure 3.4 displays the smaller (non-grand) discourses, and the processes and relations that fit under the grand discourses of old age, with their respective numbers taken from the table.

There are overlapping discourses, processes, and relations that have been classified under more than one grand discourse. One example of this occurrence is the placement of the discourse, 'old age as a burden', under both 'the medicalisation of old age', and 'old age's relationship with social welfare'. Since multiple and distinct perspectives

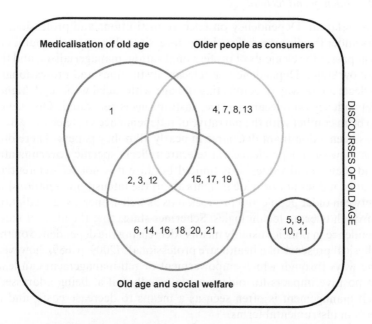

Figure 3.5 Overlapping discourses, processes, and relations between the grand discourses of old age (own illustration, 2019).

are captured within an overarching narrative (grand discourse), it has been possible for the discourses and processes identified in this chapter to be representative of more than one grand discourse. Figure 3.5 presents these classifications with the use of sets in order to clarify the overlapping elements of grand discourses and identify those discourses which exist outside the group of grand discourses.

Expanding grand discourses and other discourses of old age

Two sets of discourses and processes stand out in the allocation of the above manifestations under the grand discourses. These relate to old age discourses and old age identity in novel ways. The first set presents itself under the grand discourse of old age's relationship with social welfare, which is comprised of 'dependency on telecare institutions and professionals' (#16). The second set exists outside the three grand discourses and is comprised of: 'old age dependency as the source of unfairness between generations' (#5), 'the deserving old' (#9), 'the heroic old' (#10), and 'intergenerational debt' (#11). These four discourses reflect the theme of *social responsibility*.

Dependency and technology

The relation 'Dependency on telecare institutions and professionals' fits under the discourse of social welfare, since this grand discourse encompasses the elements of professionalisation, managerialism, and the hollow state. 'Dependency on telecare institutions and professionals' reflects a new way of connecting old age with social welfare. A higher dependency on telecare services institutions is generated. This seems to be in conflict with the narrative of independence via telecare, which has been a dominant discourse in nearly all policy papers. Therefore, the view of independence via telecare reflects specific governmental and managerial values; it is limited because it is not self-referential, that is, it does not provide insights about the intensifying relationship between older people and professionals as well as increased mediation through telecare technologies. Schermer states that the ideal of independence in policies usually means "decreasing the dependence on the physical presence of a healthcare professional" (2009, p. 689); however, the ways through which empowerment or self-management can lead to positive impacts for older people usually fail at being addressed. Self-management is often seen as a means to decrease costs, and is seen in instrumental terms.

In terms of dependencies, Guta et al.'s study (2012) also sheds light on concerns for potential future forms of telecare. The internalised surveillance through fear can become a reality in the future because adherence to treatment might be imposed by the services by reporting on those who "fail" to adhere to the government-imposed treatments (Guta et al., 2012). Reflecting on Sorell and Draper's study (2012), surveillance through care technologies will exist, regardless of whether this surveillance is chosen or imposed. It is also important to note that the freedom to choose is a technique of governmentality that makes actors accept responsibilities in the form of their own rational choices (Guta et al., 2012). The core assumption of all neoliberal analysis is the embodiment of 'rational choice' (Foucault, 2008). Telecare technologies exist in a neoliberal (post) welfare era, and the embodiment of rationality manifests itself through narratives around technologies. This can lead to viewing telecare technologies ambivalently, because the techniques of surveillance could be maintained through the technologies in the future (Guta et al., 2012).

Here it can be emphasised that the element of dependency comprises a component of surveillance embedded within it. Intensifying relationships between older people and professionals ensue in the increasing pervasiveness of telecare. This narrative of independence overshadows those processes and relations that are gradually leading

A critical enquiry into old age   105

to more dependencies and increasing surveillance. Even though the relation 'Dependency on telecare institutions and professionals' does not construct the old age identity in distinct ways, it contributes to the expansion of the social welfare grand discourse by adding new layers to it in relation to care technologies. This process is intricately linked to the narratives of personal choice and independence that confer on older people an empowered identity.

Care managerialism has been challenging dependency by appropriating the narrative of *choice* and *empowerment* in welfare discourses. I assert that care managerialism and modernisation in relation to telecare reflect only a limited version of choice, independence, and empowerment. Through processes of normalisation and standardisation, the enacted policies impose a particular form of 'choice' and 'independence' – one that is defined by the government and is laden with embedded value hierarchies from medical and economic lenses. It is worth deconstructing and investigating *from whom* or *what* exactly is the old person becoming independent (e.g. is it from their family's care and support, which the technologies are supposedly not meant to replace?), and from which range of options do they *choose*? (e.g. are the full range of options truly made available to them?).

Discourses of social responsibility

Four main discourses have emerged out of the social responsibility theme: 'old age dependency as the source of unfairness between generations' (#5), 'the deserving old' (#9), 'the heroic old' (#10), and 'intergenerational debt' (#11). Social responsibility discourses do not align with the grand discourses that have been brought together, and therefore stand outside of, but in relation to, the grand discourses. The narrative of social responsibility might be seen to be in conflict with individual responsibilities, as supported by the logics of modernisation and care management. However, this discourse can still contribute to the diffusion of modernisation logics of the neoliberal governmentality. While doing so, it redefines the identity of old age through the aforementioned discourses of unfairness between generations, deservedness of resources, and the intergenerational contract.

As Schermer (2009) reflects, care management is legitimised by the morality around distributive justice and by the 'principle of justice': "Because the society shares the medical costs, patients have a duty to do everything in their power to reduce these costs, and therefore they should be compliant" (Schermer, 2009, p. 690). This means that compliance is promoted and normalised as a moral good: older people should have the responsibility to be deserving and live their lives in healthy and productive ways; otherwise it would be seen as unfair to the next generations. The unfairness discourse is based on this distributive justice.

With social responsibility discourses, older people are defined as different and always with reference to others. This means that the old age identity has a primary referent that is the *working-age* population, through which an identity of otherness is conveyed for older people. However, the treatment of 'older people' as one distinct, singular group in these homogenising narratives fails to accommodate and address the stark disparities in living experiences among people over 65, including those of gender, ethnicity, and socio-economic standing (Fealy et al., 2012). This homogenising narrative highlights a constructed 'old age' demographic bracket as the wealthiest demographic, and places it within the 'poor working' versus 'wealthy dependent' dichotomous narrative. This means that the policies are reductively neglecting to address the stratification within this constructed 'old age' demographic, and whether there have been any shifts in this area. For example, we can put this against the reality of austerity that the support for older people has significantly declined, creating a rise in death rates amongst people aged 85 and over (Loopstra et al., 2016). Many people who have been placed into this constructed bracket of old age are living under highly precarious conditions, such as having to sell their houses for their care or living in cold homes in winter.[21]

Redefining the old age identity

My critical enquiry into policies and strategies reveals that there are various discourses and structural processes that contribute to the social positioning of older people. Old age identity cannot be separated from these discourses and structural processes. The grand discourses of old age have been continuous over a particular time frame. The discourses present within the grand discourses have been enacted in various ways in policies and strategies. If we reflect back on Weedon's definition of identity,

> as a limited and temporary fixing for the individual of a particular mode of subjectivity (...) to curtail the plural possibilities of subjectivity inherent in the wider discursive field and to give individuals a singular sense of who they are and where they belong,
> (2004, p. 19)

this kind of singular sense of being has been highly echoed in my analysis.

Modern interventions of the state give life to the population with the propagation of health and longevity, and the categorisations of older people can serve such functions as targeting public resources to meet particular needs in this population. While being cognisant of this, however, the state government and social services institutions also constrain this population with the continuous monitoring of life; the same categorisations can have negative consequences too, such as positioning older people as passive, dependent, and in need of care. For example, the analysis of policies revealed that 'older people' are categorised as a homogenised group with reference to their current 'inactivity' (as opposed to the productivity of working-age people), and to their chronological age. By implication, this constitutes a uniform identity of dependency.

Furthermore, the medicalisation of bodies constitutes new forms of power/knowledge relations by which normal/abnormal, and illness/ health are defined (Foucault, 1994b). The most powerful and normalised discourses – those that have the most productive social effects – depend on the *regime of truth*, on the assumption that their knowledge is true (Rose, G., 2001). With the categorisation of the individual (by scientific classifications and dividing practices), the individual becomes a carrier of meaning and of an identity (Dagg and Haugaard, 2016). The policies analysed in this chapter are the "validator of that subject identity" which "impose upon [individuals] a form of control" (ibid., p. 397). The type of governmentalisation identified within old age and telecare related policies makes "social and personal consequences of [old age] an object of political concern", and renders older people "knowable, calculable and thereby amenable to various strategies of intervention" (Wahlberg and Rose, 2015, p. 1).

The grand discourses and other discourses of old age reflect the logics and rationalities of the current regime of truth. Discourses are "socially constitutive as well as socially conditioned – [they] constitute situations, objects of knowledge, and the social identities of and relationship between people and groups of people" (Fairclough and Wodak, 1997, p. 258). Discourses are socially consequential because they can help to sustain the status quo. In this book, those discourses that have been enacting the grand discourses of old age have been identified. In addition to this, I reflected on the disruption of certain discourses and highlighted significant old age discourses that have not historically existed as part of the grand narratives.

Old age identity is the combination of these continuous and disrupted discourses and grand discourses. Most discourses of old age – as expressed through telecare policies – place older people outside of the society and assume homogeneity of their identities. Representing older people as the unproductive population, as a risk, and as deserving of tax-funded benefits constructs an identity of dependence, which supports yet another identity: older people as 'different than', 'distinct from', or 'other to'. In the construction of this present identity of otherness, discontinuities have been observed between past and present identities of older people. For example, there was no reference to older people's *working-age* years – apart from declaring older people as wartime heroes; and a discourse of opposition was used in policies: working-age versus older people.

The 'social welfare' grand discourse of old age has been expanded with the addition of technology relations, and the 'choice' and 'empowerment' narratives have been disrupted. This is because the independence narrative has been overshadowing the increase of certain dependencies and the intensifying gaze over older people. The freedom to choose has been defined as a technique of governmentality that transfers responsibilities over older people through their own rational choices (Guta et al., 2012). The embodiment of 'rational choice' was defined as a central assumption of neoliberal governance (Foucault, 2008). Therefore, the narratives of choice and empowerment are revealed as an apparatus of surveillance.

On the other hand, a new cluster of old age discourses were found to have implications on the identity of old age alongside the historical constructions of identity via grand discourses. Social responsibility discourses demonstrated that the old age identity is constructed in ambivalent ways. Because the apparatuses of modernisation and care management reflect the welfare state's transforming neoliberal values and logics – such as 'politics of participation' (Powell and Biggs, 2000), self-responsibility, and individualisation – I identified social responsibility as a shifting discourse, whose continuity still manifests in policies. This leads us to the conclusion that social responsibility discourse is a vehicle that appeals to traditional community values, while also carrying forward the practices of intervention in older people's lives.

As a powerful narrative, social responsibility supports the conflicting logics and processes of social care modernisation and care management, and it reveals the morality around a system of 'distributive justice' (Schermer, 2009), whilst appealing to community values. One discourse constitutes old age dependency as a source of unfairness towards younger generations (based on the implied principle of distributive justice); the other two discourses construct the old age identity as deserving of the younger generations' help due to intergenerational debt. In these conflicting discourses, a commonality is identified: older people are always defined with reference to younger age groups.

Moreover, some narratives present in policies reflect certain misleading positions about old age by presenting it as a homogeneous identity. I argue that policies are reductively neglecting to address the stratification within the constructed 'old age' demographic. The homogenisation of old age can distract from highly pertinent issues, such as the realities of precarious conditions that old people live with, and the increasing stratification and gap between poorer and better-off members of all age demographics in the UK.[22]

The identity constructions in relation to telecare therefore separate old age from the rest of the population, and institutionalise the distinctions between older people and mainstream society. These identities are constructed through placing older people outside of society – as secondary, peripheral, dependent – and as discontinuous in terms of their past and present identities. The construction of these identities matters for older people because: (1) certain forms of governance are formed that describe, judge, measure, and compare by "imposing new delimitations on them" (Foucault, 1977, p. 184), and (2) this leads to *technologies of the self* (Foucault, 1982) and *looping effects* (Hacking, 1995). With the discourses and identities acknowledged in this chapter, it can be said that older people comprise a distinct *human kind*, and that older people turn themselves into subjects of old age too. The classifications by scientific disciplines (those that are referred to in policies) are intricately linked with how older people construct their own selves. Therefore, the dominant old age identities and powerful discourses that emerged from policies are likely to produce social effects; because socially positioning older people is intricately linked with older people constructing their own selves.

Notes

1 In this book, 'NHS' mainly refers to NHS England.
2 New Labour is a period of history of the British Labour Party from the middle of 1990s until 2010 under the governments of Tony Blair and Gordon Brown. The name comes from a conference slogan, 'New Labour, New Life for Britain', which was used by the party in 1990s.
3 Primary care is the first point of contact for people in need of health care, and is provided by professionals such as GPs, dentists, pharmacists, and eye health professionals (NHS Providers, 2018).
4 Secondary care is referred to as the 'hospital and community care'. It can "either be planned care such as a cataract operation, or urgent and emergency care such as treatment for a fracture" (NHS Providers, 2018).
5 "The Royal Commission on Long Term Care for the Elderly was appointed in December 1997 to examine the short- and long-term options for a sustainable system of funding of long-term care for elderly people,

110 *A critical enquiry into old age*

both in their homes and other settings" (National Archives, 2016). In 1999, a grand report was published by the commission, and many recommendations were put forward for the government about the future of care, including the proposal for free personal care. The Royal Commission has not been active since; however, in the following decades, their proposals kept being used as a substantial foundation for political discussions around social care.

6 This was the largest charity for older people until 2009, before the two charities, Age Concern England and Help the Aged, merged and formed the current Age UK.
7 "The Housing Corporation was the non-departmental public body that funded new affordable housing and regulated housing associations in England. It was abolished in 2008 with its responsibilities being split between the Homes and Communities Agency and the Tenant Services Authority" (GOV.UK, 2008).
8 "The IGP programme is a revenue grant administered by the Housing Corporation to encourage the development and testing of new ideas and proposals and to generate and promote good practice in the delivery of housing services within the housing association sector" (UK Housing, 2007).
9 England's largest not-for-profit provider of housing and care for people aged 55 and over.
10 Assistive technology is "any device or system that allows an individual to perform a task that they would otherwise be unable to do, or increases the ease and safety with which the task can be performed" (Royal Commission on Long Term Care, 1999).
11 "Adult social care – the provision of support and personal care (as opposed to treatment) to meet needs arising from illness, disability or old age – is funded by the Department for Communities and Local Government (DCLG) and managed through local authorities" (Institute for Government, 2017).
12 Telecare Services Association (TSA) is a non-profit organisation that influences national policy, sets standards for the industry, advises on commissioning and procurement, organises events, and offers relevant training (TSA, 2017a). Several organisations that provide telecare products or services go under an audit for the TSA's Quality Standards Framework (QSF) accreditation. After being the primary framework in the accreditation of telecare services in the UK since 2013, TSA's QSF was publicly endorsed in 2017 by the Parliamentary under Secretary of State for Community Health and Care (TSA, 2017b).
13 The full reference list of all documents can be accessed in the Appendices.
14 The Think Tank Panel met in 2016 to consider recent developments in the adoption of care technologies in the UK, and to consult on the TSA's new 'Technology Roadmap' to guide the industry through changes (TSA, 2016a, 2016b).
15 "Being person-centred is about focusing care on the needs of individual. Ensuring that people's preferences, needs and values guide clinical decisions, and providing care that is respectful of and responsive to them" (Health Education England, 2016).

16 The Big Care Debate consultation followed the government's green paper Shaping the Future of Care Together (HM Government, 2009), which was published in July 2009, and it ran until November 2009. The government received 28,000 consultation responses and held 37 events around the country (House of Commons Health Committee, 2010).
17 A full list of these visual exhibits can be accessed in the Appendices section.
18 The 'Easy Read' versions of government documents serve the purpose of creating an accessible way to engage with and inform the public. Based on the requirements by Equality Act 2000, government organisations are bound to ensure that their services and publications are accessible to disabled people, after which large print and Easy Read versions became more common (National Archives, 2017).
19 In 2015–2016, there were over 1.8 million requests for social care services in England from new clients. 72 per cent of these were reported to be from clients aged 65 and over (Adult Social Care Team – NHS Digital, 2016).
20 "The enormous sacrifices of the wartime generation demanded that there had to be an ambitious programme for quality healthcare, alongside economic reconstruction. Now that same generation is owed a further debt of dignity: to receive care and to stay in their homes as long as possible" (HM Government, 2010, p. 2).
21 Age UK (2015) has reported that there have been 2.5 million avoidable deaths among older people in England and Wales due to the winter cold over the last 60 years. High energy bills are identified to be one of the primary causes of the problem.
22 "As well as average wealth levels, there are also big differences in how equally wealth is distributed within generations (...) Gaps in net financial wealth between poorer and better-off members of older cohorts are very large and have risen in recent years" (Intergenerational Commission, 2017, p. 6).

4 Conclusions and future directions

In this book, I investigated and revealed the old age discourses embedded within care policies and strategies relevant to telecare, which were found to be connected to and indicative of wider trends and structural relations. The problematisation of old age via care policies provides the conditions in which telecare technologies are offered as solutions to the "old age problem". However, telecare technologies are not socially vacuous solutions, that is to say, solutions that are neutral and devoid of values and politics; because various dominant normalisations and rationalisations of governmentality are embedded in the legitimisation and implementation of telecare technologies.

It is important to study telecare technologies because of the increasing expenditure on these technologies and the intensifying legitimisation processes by consecutive governments in the UK. It is also necessary to examine these technologies always within their wider political, economic, and social domains. The discursive policies around telecare reflect those changes in the wider context; they also have social consequences on the lives of older people, such as the means through which they access services and funding, their negotiation with the gatekeepers to services, the frequency and quality of their relationship with health and social care professionals and their support groups, their well-being and mental health, and so on.

With the analysis of policies, I revealed the (1) discourses that enact the grand discourses of old age, (2) new processes and relations in the lives of older people in relation to telecare, and (3) those discourses that overshadow certain narratives and relations. These processes and relations – namely, *modernisation of care services* and *care managerialism* – represent dominant structures within the domain of neoliberal economic policies, and they have marked effects on old age discourses. Narratives about old age were found in many cases to be dissonant, and in some cases arguably misleading and reductive in their

Conclusions 113

depiction of older people as a somehow fixed, stable, homogeneous, and singular group, as opposed to a reference to a fluid state of being (age) that artificially links a diverse range of people – highly stratified in terms of their lifestyles, values, culture, socio-economic conditions, etc. I concluded that the identity construction of old age in relation to telecare separates old age from the rest of the population, and positions them as dependent and as discontinuous in terms of their past and present identities. This positioning of older people as an 'other to' mainstream society constitutes a redefined identity of old age.

The analysis conducted captures a *snapshot* of the early intervention period of the state government and local authorities in the wider deployment of telecare technologies. Since the dominant logic and rationalities embedded in telecare technologies are the biased carriers of meanings about old age, this snapshot presents those narratives surrounding, and enabled by, telecare. Identities present a limited and temporary fixing for individuals (Weedon, 2004); therefore, the use of this metaphor – taking a snapshot – mirrors the understanding of how identities work.

It is worthwhile to remember again that modern interventions of the state governments are planned to give life to the population with the propagation of improved health and longevity, and that categorising older people can serve such functions in targeting public resources to meet particular needs in the population. Telecare is becoming embedded into the routines of everyday life for many users, and this is not solely a product of a governmental agenda. The practical value of telecare is increasing due to technological developments, which translates into cheaper and better equipment. In the era of neoliberal governmentality, recognising the individualising effects of social care reforms would be essential, because individual responsibilities over social responsibilities are becoming a reality. This indicates a change in social relationships and interactions, as well as a rise in difficulties such as loneliness and social isolation. Therefore, telecare can be a 'solution' in several respects, and it can indeed empower its users; however, the less favourable social effects of telecare should also be made visible.

I critically approach the issue that the governments, as well as giving life to the population, also constrain older people with the construction of knowledge on old age through telecare. The same governmental categorisations that serve specific functions can also have other less desirable consequences on social life by giving individuals "a singular sense of who they are and where they belong" (Weedon, 2004, p. 19). This homogenisation can erase the complexity of needs, capabilities, dispositions, and preferences in individual lives whilst obscuring highly pertinent social issues, such as gaps in financial wealth, especially of older-age cohorts.

Policy recommendations

Public policy papers offer a window on governmental values in the wider context of political, social, and economic processes. At the same time, they can be important vehicles in the formation of public opinion. I demonstrated that: (a) the language in policy discourses constructs old age in particular ways through the selective filtering or selective construction of knowledge (mainly economic and statistical) and (b) the language of policies is rarely neutral. Because of this constitutive power, the onus is on the governments in the way they represent older people or any other particular social group.

Apart from the social responsibility discourse, it has been the case that the policies and the strategies identified do not reflect older people's contributions to the enrichment of society. Even when the theme of social responsibility is laid out in policies, the discourse is constructed upon older people being deserving/undeserving based on wartime sacrifices and their past contributions to society. It is recommended that "older people should be conducted with reference to their role as fully contributing members of society and not as a social group outside of mainstream society" (NCPOP, 2009, p. 28). Labelling and referencing older people at the level of national policies and strategies should undergo a careful consideration to avoid implying homogeneity of this group with reference to their capabilities, socio-economic status, and social care needs.

Further research

Telecare technologies are powerful mediators of discourses and are bound to be an even more significant part of older people's lives in the near future. In the UK, "an ageing population met with the reduction of social care funding" (Cook et al., 2018, p. 1912) has been leading to a reduction in support that is available to older people. The innovative telecare technologies are viewed as a viable way to support older people, and there are more recent studies in various fields that have been conducted on such topics as barriers to the adoption of telecare technologies, factors that influence the decision to adopt telecare, factors that are predictive of its continued use, and the importance of context in the implementation and adoption of telecare (Bozan et al., 2016; Cook et al., 2016; Hsu et al., 2016; Yusif et al., 2016; Berge, 2017; Hamblin et al., 2017; Cook et al., 2018). Besides academic studies, research is carried out by the UK and EU public bodies, which evaluate the state of telecare and devise new strategies for improvement (JAseHN EU, 2017; King's Fund, 2018; TSA, 2018). The ongoing academic and public engagement with these technologies reflects that there are still noteworthy consequences, challenges, concerns, and debates surrounding telecare, which makes telecare technologies significantly relevant in terms of the discourses they may mediate.

In this book, it has been revealed that telecare information systems are driven by certain powerful – and sometimes conflicting – rationalities and discourses about old age. The old age identity constructed upon these discourses does not only socially position older people for others, but also constitutes an own sense of identity for older people. This is why it is imperative to suggest further research that is concerned with the *self-subjectification* practices (the third mode of objectification). More reflection upon the everyday practices of older people with telecare and on the consequences of *looping effects* can add important insights to the full circle of modes of objectification.

Finally, one demographic that has been missing or that was overshadowed from policies and strategies has been individuals with disabilities. Older people with disabilities have the highest prevalence of disability within their age group (65 and over) compared to other age groups, yet people with disabilities from other age groups are overall higher in number.[1] The policies analysed in this book – about housing, carers, telecare, and other social care issues – have mainly focussed on old age. As further research, it would be a pertinent endeavour to investigate those narratives in care policies that target people with disabilities, and to map a genealogy of the disabled identity in relation to technological care.

Note

1 The prevalence of disability rises with age, although there are more people with disabilities who are below state pension age. "In 2012/2013, 7% of children were disabled (0.9 million), compared to 16% of adults of working age (6.1 million), and 43% of adults over state pension age (5.1 million)" (Papworth Trust, 2016, p. 8).

References

3ML. (2012). About 3ML. http://3millionlives.co.uk/about-3ml

3ML. (2013). 3millionlives – Enabling change to benefit patients and carers. Retrieved April 27, 2013 from https://web.archive.org/web/20140705032311/http://3millionlives.co.uk/wp-content/uploads/2013/03/3ml-news-release-22-March-2013.pdf.

Adass/Association of Directors of Adult Social Services. (2017). Adass budget survey – 2017. https://www.adass.org.uk/media/5994/adass-budget-survey-report-2017.pdf

Adult Social Care Team-NHS Digital. (2016). Community care statistics, social services activity, England, 2015–16. https://digital.nhs.uk/data-and-information/publications/statistical/community-care-statistics-social-services-activity/community-care-statistics-social-services-activity-england-2015-16

Age Concern. (1998). *A Guide to the Debate of the Age – Your Say in the Future*. Age Concern England, London.

Age UK. (2015). Highest excess winter deaths this century. https://www.ageuk.org.uk/latest-news/archive/highest-excess-winter-deaths-this-century/

Age UK. (2017). Changes to the way you pay for residential care. https://www.ageuk.org.uk/information-advice/care/social-care-and-support-where-to-start/paying-for-care-support/changes-to-the-way-you-pay-for-residential-care/

Ainsworth, S., and Hardy, C. (2007). The construction of the older worker: Privilege, paradox and policy. *Discourse & Communication*, 1(3), 267–285.

Alvarez, R. (2005). Taking a critical linguistic turn: Using critical discourse analysis for the study of information systems. In D. Howcroft and E. M. Trauth (eds.), *Handbook of Critical Information Systems Research: Theory and Application*, pp. 104–122. Edward Elgar, Cheltenham.

Alvesson, M., and Sköldberg, K. (2009). *Reflexive Methodology: New Vistas for Qualitative Research*. SAGE, London.

Alzheimer Society. (2011). The dementia tax 2011-Alzheimer's society public policy report, (June 2011). https://www.alzheimers.org.uk/sites/default/files/migrate/downloads/dementia_tax_report_2011.pdf

References

Audit Commission. (2004). Older people: Implementing telecare. Retrieved June 16, 2014 from http://www.auditcommission.gov.uk/reports/NATIONAL-REPORT.asp?CategoryID=&ProdID=BDBE0111-764C-44a4-8A66-1CB25D 6974A4.
Avgerou, C. (2000). Information systems: What sort of science is it? *Omega*, 28(5), 567–579.
Avgerou, C. (2002). *Information Systems and Global Diversity*. Oxford University Press, Oxford.
Avgerou, C., and McGrath, K. (2005). Rationalities and emotions in IS innovation. In D. Howcroft and E. M. Trauth (eds.), *Handbook of Critical Information Systems Research: Theory and Application*, pp. 299–324. Edward Elgar, Cheltenham.
Bauman, Z. (2000). *Liquid Modernity*. Polity Press, Cambridge.
BBC News. (2005). NHS use of private sector to rise. http://news.bbc.co.uk/1/hi/health/4542009.stm
BBH / Building Better Healthcare. (2014). Shropshire council partners with Tunstall advisory service for assistive technology programme. https://www.buildingbetterhealthcare.co.uk/news/article_page/Shropshire_Council_partners_with_Tunstall_Advisory_Service_for_assistive_technology_programme/101603
Beck, U. (1992). *Risk Society*. Sage, London.
Beck, U. (2007). Beyond class and nation: Reframing social inequalities in a globalizing world. *British Journal of Sociology*, 58(4), 679–705.
Beck, U., Giddens, A., and Lash, S. (1994). *Reflexive Modernization – Politics, Tradition and Aesthetics in Modern Social Order*. Polity Press, Cambridge.
Berge, M. S. (2017). Telecare – Where, when, why and for whom does it work? A realist evaluation of a Norwegian project. *Journal of Rehabilitation and Assistive Technologies Engineering*, 4, 1–10.
Biggs, S. (2001). Toward critical narrativity stories of aging in contemporary social policy. *Journal of Aging Studies*, 15(4), 303–316.
Biggs, S., and Powell, J. L. (1999). Surveillance and elder abuse: The rationalities and technologies of community care. *Journal of Contemporary Health*, 4(1), 43–49.
Biggs, S., and Powell, J. L. (2001). A Foucauldian analysis of old age and the power of social welfare. *Journal of Aging & Social Policy*, 12(2), 93–112.
Bonacker, T. (2006). What do we have in common? Modernity and the paradoxes of postnational integration. *Studies in Social and Political Thought*, 10, 73–97.
Bozan, K., Parker, K., and Davey, B. (2016). *A Closer Look at the Social Influence Construct in the UTAUT Model: An Institutional Theory Based Approach to Investigate Health IT Adoption Patterns of the Elderly*. In Proceedings of the 2016 49th Hawaii International Conference on System Sciences (HICSS '16). IEEE Computer Society, Washington, DC, USA, 3105–3114.
Brooke, C. (2002). What does it mean to be 'critical' in IS research? *Journal of Information Technology*, 17, 49–57.
Bryman, A. (2012). *Social Research Methods*. Oxford University Press, New York.

Care UK. (2017). Our history. http://www.careukgroup.com/about-us/our-history

Carers UK. (2012). Carers and telecare. https://www.carersuk.org/for-professionals/policy/policy-library?task=download&file=policy_file&id=3501

Carr, N. (2008). The great unbundling. In N. Carr (ed.), *The Big Switch: Rewiring the World from Edison to Google*, pp. 149–167. W.W. Norton and Company, New York.

Cartwright, M., Hirani, S. P., Rixon, L., Beynon, M., Doll, H., Bower, P., Bardsley, M., Steventon, A., Knapp, M., Henderson, C., Rogers, A., Sanders, C., Fitzpatrick, R., Barlow, J., and Newman, S. P. (2013). Effect of telehealth on quality of life and psychological outcomes over 12 months (Whole Systems Demonstrator telehealth questionnaire study): Nested study of patient reported outcomes in a pragmatic, cluster randomised controlled trial. *BMJ*, 346, 1–20.

CCACE / Centre for Cognitive Ageing and Cognitive Epidemiology. (2011). Systematic reviews and meta-analyses: A step-by-step guide. https://www.ccace.ed.ac.uk/research/software-resources/systematic-reviews-and-meta-analyses

Cecez-Kecmanovic, D. (2005). Basic assumptions of the critical research perspectives in information systems. In D. Howcroft and E. M. Trauth (eds.), *Handbook of Critical Information Systems Research: Theory and Application*, pp. 19–46. Edward Elgar, Cheltenham.

Commission on the Future of Health and Social Care in England. (2014). The UK private health market. https://www.kingsfund.org.uk/sites/default/files/media/commission-appendix-uk-private-health-market.pdf

Community Care. (2002). Better government for older people network. http://www.communitycare.co.uk/2002/08/06/better-government-for-older-people-network/

Cook, E. J., Randhawa, G., Guppy, A., Sharp, C., Barton, G., Bateman, A., and Crawford-White, J. (2018). Exploring factors that impact the decision to use assistive telecare: Perspectives of family care-givers of older people in the United Kingdom. *Ageing and Society*, 38(9), 1912–1932.

Cook, E. J., Randhawa, G., Sharp, C., Ali, N., Guppy, A., Barton, G., Bateman, A., and Crawford-White, J. (2016). Exploring the factors that influence the decision to adopt and engage with an integrated assistive telehealth and telecare service in Cambridgeshire, UK: A nested qualitative study of patient 'users' and 'non-users'. *BMC Health Services Research*, 16, 137.

Cottam, R. (1954). Growing old. In *Living Longer: Some Social Aspects of the Problem of Old Age*. The National Council of Social Service, London.

Curry, R. G., Tinoco, M. T., and Wardle, D. (2002). The use of Information and Communication Technology (ICT) to support independent living for older and disabled people. http://www.rehabtool.com/forum/discussions/ictuk02.pdf

References

Dagg, J., and Haugaard, M. (2016). The performance of subject positions, power, and identity: A case of refugee recognition. *European Journal of Cultural and Political Sociology*, 3(4), 392–425.

Deetz, S. (1992). *Democracy in an Age of Corporate Colonization: Developments in Communication and the Politics of Everyday Life*. State University of New York Press, Albany.

Dews, P. (1984). Power and subjectivity in Foucault. *New Left Review*, 144, 72–95.

Diaz-Bone, R., Bührmann, A. D., Gutiérrez Rodríguez, E., Schneider, W., Kendall, G., and Tirado, F. (2007). The field of Foucaultian discourse analysis: Structures, developments and perspectives. *Forum: Qualitative Social Research*, 8(2), 1–21.

Dorset Council. (2019). Telecare choice. https://www.dorsetcouncil.gov.uk/care-and-support-for-adults/service-directory/telecare-choice.aspx#/

Eisenstadt, S. (2000). Multiple modernities. *Journal of the American Academy of Arts and Science*, 129(1), 1–29.

Ermisch, J. (1990). *Fewer Babies, Longer Lives*. Joseph Rowntree Foundation, York.

Estes, C., and Linkins, K. W. (1997). Devolution and aging policy: Racing to the bottom in long-term care. *International Journal of Health Services*, 27(3), 427–442.

Fairclough, N. (1989). *Language and Power*. Longman, Harlow.

Fairclough, N. (1995). *Critical Discourse Analysis*. Longman, London.

Fairclough, N. (2010). *Critical Discourse Analysis: The Critical Study of Language*. Routledge, London.

Fairclough, N., and Wodak, R. (1997). Critical discourse analysis. In T. A. van Dijk, (ed.), *Discourse as Social Interaction: Discourse Studies: A Multidisciplinary Introduction*, vol. 2, pp. 258–284. SAGE, London.

Fealy, G., McNamara, M., Treacy, M. P., and Lyons, I. (2012). Constructing ageing and age identities: A case study of newspaper discourses. *Ageing & Society*, 31, 85–102.

Featherstone, M. (1987). Leisure, symbolic power and the life course. In D. Jary, S. Home, and A. Tomlinson (eds.), *Sport, Leisure and Social Relations*, pp. 113–138. Routledge, London.

Featherstone, M., and Hepworth, M. (1989). Ageing and old age: Reflections on the postmodern life course. In B. Bytheway, T. Keil, P. Allat, and A. Bryman (eds.), *Becoming and Being Old*, pp. 143–157. Sage, London.

Featherstone, M., and Wernick, A. (1995). *Images of Aging: Cultural Representations of Later Life*. Routledge, London.

Feenberg, A. (2003). Background texts and applications – "Critical theory of technology." https://www.sfu.ca/~andrewf/background_applications.html

Fernandez, J. L., Snell, T., and Wistow, G. (2013). Changes in the patterns of social care provision in England: 2005/6 to 2012/13. Personal Social Services Research Unit Discussion Paper 2867. December 2013. https://www.pssru.ac.uk/pub/dp2867.pdf

Foucault, M. (1967). On the ways of writing history. In J. D. Faubion (ed.), *Aesthetics, Method and Epistemology* (The Essential Works of Michel Foucault 1954–1984, vol. 2), pp. 279–295. Penguin, Middlesex.

Foucault, M. (1969). *L'archéologie du savoir.* Gallimard, Paris. Translated as *The Archaeology of Knowledge.* Allan Sheridan (trans.), Harper and Row, New York.

Foucault, M. (1970). *L'Ordre du Discours.* Éditions Gallimard, Paris.

Foucault, M. (1975). *The Birth of the Clinic.* Vintage Books, New York.

Foucault, M. (1977). *Discipline and Punish: The Birth of the Prison.* Tavistock, London.

Foucault, M. (1980a). *The History of Sexuality. Vol.1: An Introduction.* Vintage Books, New York.

Foucault, M. (1980b). Power/*Knowledge: Selected Interviews and Other Writings 1972–1977.* Pantheon Books, New York.

Foucault, M. (1982). The subject and power. *Critical Inquiry*, 8(4), 777–795.

Foucault, M. (1985). *The History of Sexuality. Vol.2: The Use of Pleasure.* Vintage Books, New York.

Foucault, M. (1986). *The History of Sexuality. Vol.3: The Care of the Self.* Vintage Books, New York.

Foucault, M. (1991). Governmentality. In G. Burchell, C. Gordon, and P. Miller (eds.), *The Foucault Effect: Studies in Governmentality*, pp. 87–104. Harvester Wheatsheaf, Hemel Hempstead.

Foucault, M. (1993). About the beginning of the hermeneutics of the self. *Political Theory*, 21, 198–227.

Foucault, M. (1994a). The ethic of care for the self as a practice of freedom: An interview with Michel Foucault. In J. Bernauer and D. Rasmussen (eds.), *The Final Foucault*, pp. 1–20. MIT Press, Cambridge.

Foucault, M. (1994b). *The Order of Things: An Archaeology of the Human Sciences.* Vintage Books, New York.

Foucault, M. (1996). *Foucault Live: Interviews, 1961–1984.* S. Lotringer (ed.), Semiotext(e), New York.

Foucault, M. (1997). On the genealogy of ethics: An overview of work in progress. In P. Rabinow (ed.), *Ethics, Subjectivity and Truth: The Essential Works*, pp. 253–280. Penguin Press, London.

Foucault, M. (2008). *The Birth of Biopolitics: Lectures at the Collège de France, 1978–79.* G. Burchell (trans.), Palgrave Macmillan, New York.

Foucault, M., and Sennett, R. (1982). Sexuality and solitude. *Humanities in Review*, 1, 3–21.

Fukuyama, F. (1996). *Trust: The Social Virtues and the Creation of Prosperity.* Simon and Schuster, New York.

Full Fact. (2017). What is the "dementia tax"? https://fullfact.org/health/what-dementia-tax/

Giaschi, P. (2000). Gender positioning in education: A critical image analysis of ESL texts. *TESL Canada Journal*, 18(1), 32–46.

Giddens, A. (1991). *Modernity and Self-Identity.* Polity Press, Oxford.

Gilleard, C., and Higgs, P. (2014). *Ageing, Corporeality and Embodiment.* Anthem Press, London.

References

Goldenberg, M. J. (2006). On evidence and evidence-based medicine: Lessons from the philosophy of science. *Social Science and Medicine (1982)*, 62(11), 2621–2632.

GOV.UK. (2008). Housing corporation. https://www.gov.uk/government/organisations/housing-corporation

Greenhalgh, T. (2012). Whole system demonstrator trial: Policy, politics, and publication ethics. *BMJ*, 345, 5280.

Guta, A., Gagnon, M., and Jacob, J. D. (2012). Using Foucault to recast the telecare debate. *The American Journal of Bioethics*, 12(9), 57–59.

Habermas, J. (1971). *Knowledge and Human Interests*. Heinemann, London.

Hacking, I. (1995). The looping effects of human kinds. In D. Sperber, D. Premack, and A. J. Premack (eds.), *Causal Cognition: A Multidisciplinary Debate*, pp. 351–394. Oxford University Press, New York.

Hacking, I. (1999). *The Social Construction of What?* Harvard University Press, Cambridge.

Hamblin, K., Yeandle, S., and Fry, G. (2017). Researching telecare: The importance of context. *Journal of Enabling Technologies*, 11(3), 75–84.

Harvey, D. (2007). *A Brief History of Neoliberalism*. Oxford University Press, New York.

Hastings, A., Bailey, N., Bramley, G., Gannon, M., and Watkins, D. (2015). The cost of the cuts: The impact on local government and poorer communities. Joseph Rowntree Foundation Report, (March), 5–127.

Health Education England. (2016). Person-centred care. https://www.hee.nhs.uk/our-work/person-centred-care

Henderson, C., Knapp, M., Beecham, J., Hirani, S. P., Cartwright, M., Rixon, L., Beynon, M., Rogers, A., Power, P., Doll, H., Fitzpatrick, R., Steventon, A., Bardsley, M., Hendy, J., and Newman, S. P. (2013). Cost effectiveness of telehealth for patients with long term conditions (Whole Systems Demonstrator telehealth questionnaire study): Nested economic evaluation in a pragmatic, cluster randomised controlled trial. *BMJ*, 346, 1035, 1–19.

Henderson, C., Knapp, M., Fernández, J. L., Beecham, J., Hirani, S. P., Beynon, M., Cartwright, M., Rixon, L., Doll, H., Bower, P., Steventon, A., Rogers, A., Fitzpatrick, R., Barlow, J., Bardsley, M., and Newman, S. P. (2014). Cost-effectiveness of telecare for people with social care needs: The whole systems demonstrator cluster randomised trial. *Age and Ageing*, 43(6), 794–800.

Hirani, S. P., Beynon, M., Cartwright, M., Rixon, L., Doll, H., Henderson, C., Bardsley, M., Steventon, A., Knapp, M., Rogers, A., Bower, P., Sanders, C., Fitzpatrick, R., Hendy, J., and Newman, S. P. (2013). The effect of telecare on the quality of life and psychological well-being of elderly recipients of social care over a 12-month period: The Whole Systems Demonstrator cluster randomised trial. *Age and Ageing*, 43(3), 334–341.

Hirst, P. (1981). The genesis of the social. *Politics and Power*, 3, 67–82.

History and Policy. (2007). Trade unions and the law - History and a way forward? http://www.historyandpolicy.org/policy-papers/papers/trade-unions-and-the-law-history-and-a-way-forward

House of Commons Health Committee. (2010). Social care: Third report of session 2009–10, vol. 1. House of Commons, London.
House of Commons Library. (2012). NHS funding and expenditure. http://www.nhshistory.net/parlymoney.pdf
Howarth, D. (1998). Discourse theory and political analysis. In E. Scarbrough and E. Tanenbaum (eds.), *Research Strategies in Social Sciences: A Guide to New Approaches*, pp. 268–293. Oxford University Press, New York.
Hsu, Y. C., Tsai, C. H., Kuo, Y. M., Lien, and Ya-Hui, B. (2016). Telecare services for elderly: Predictive factors of continued use intention. *The Open Biomedical Engineering Journal*, 10, 82–90.
Humphreys, A. (2006). The consumer as Foucauldian "object of knowledge." *Social Science Computer Review*, 24(3), 296–309.
IFS / The Institute for Fiscal Studies. (2017). Budget 2017: IFS says Britain facing 'third parliament of austerity' after 2020. https://www.theguardian.com/politics/blog/live/2017/mar/09/circumstances-have-moved-on-hammond-defends-breaking-tory-manifesto-promise-on-nics-politics-live
Intergenerational Commission. (2017). The generation of wealth: Asset accumulation across and within cohorts. https://www.resolutionfoundation.org/app/uploads/2017/06/Wealth.pdf
Institute for Government. (2017). Adult social care. https://www.instituteforgovernment.org.uk/publication/performance-tracker-autumn-2017/health-and-social-care/adult-social-care
Irvine, E. (1954). Research into problem families. *British Journal of Psychiatric Social Work*, 9, 24–33.
Janks, H. (1997). Critical discourse analysis as a research tool. *Discourse: Studies in the Cultural Politics of Education*, 18(3), 329–342.
JAseHN EU / Joint Action to Support the eHealth Network EU. (2017). Report on EU state of play on telemedicine services and uptake recommendations. https://ec.europa.eu/health/sites/health/files/ehealth/docs/ev_20171128_co09_en.pdf
Jones, C. (1983). *State Social Work and the Working Class.* Macmillan, London.
Katz, S. (1996). *Disciplining Old Age: The Formation of Gerontological Knowledge.* University Press of Virginia, Charlottesville.
Katz, S. (2010). Sociocultural perspectives on ageing bodies (Chapter 27). In D. Dannefer and C. Phillipson (eds.), *The SAGE Handbook of Social Gerontology.* Sage Publications, London.
Katz, S., and Marshall, B. L. (2004). Is the functional "normal"? Aging, sexuality and the bio-marking of successful living. *History of the Human Sciences*, 17(1), 53–75.
King's Fund. (2018). Key challenges facing the adult social care sector in England. September 2018. https://www.kingsfund.org.uk/sites/default/files/2018-12/Key-challenges-facing-the-adult-social-care-sector-in-England.pdf
King's Fund and Nuffield Trust. (2016). Social care for older people: Home truths. September 2016. https://www.kingsfund.org.uk/sites/default/files/

field/field_publication_file/Social_care_older_people_Kings_Fund_Sep_2016.pdf
Klecun, E. (2004). Conducting critical research in information systems: Can actor-network theory help? In B. Kaplan, D. P. Truex, D. Wastell, A. T. Wood-Harper, and J. I. DeGross (eds.), *Information Systems Research: Relevant Theory and Informed Practice*, pp. 259–274. Springer US, New York.
Klecun, E. (2005). Competing rationalities: A critical study of telehealth in the UK. In D. Howcroft and E. M. Trauth (eds.), *Handbook of Critical Information Systems Research: Theory and Application*, pp. 388–416. Edward Elgar, Cheltenham.
Klecun, E. (2016). Transforming healthcare: Policy discourses of ICT and patient-centred care. *European Journal of Information Systems*, 25(1), 64–76.
Klecun-Dabrowska, E. (2003). Telehealth in the UK: A critical perspective. *Electronic Journal of Business Research Methods*, 2(1), 37–45.
Klecun-Dabrowska, E., and Cornford, T. (2000). Telehealth acquires meanings: Information and communication technologies within health policy. *Info Systems Journal*, 10, 41–63.
Klecun-Dabrowska, E., and Cornford, T. (2002). *The organising vision of telehealth*. In ECIS. Gdansk, Poland, 44, 1206–1217.
Lash, S. (1994). Reflexivity and its doubles: Structures, aesthetics, community. In U. Beck, A. Giddens, and S. Lash (eds.), *Reflexive Modernisation*. Polity, Cambridge.
Leicestershire County Council. (2019). Telecare choice. https://www.leicestershire.gov.uk/popular-now/directories/information-and-support-directory/telecare-choice
Leonard, P. (1997). *Postmodern Welfare*. Sage, London.
Lim, M. (2012). The personalisation of English adult social care: Political programmes and technologies of government (LSE Lecture AC500-22 February 2012).
Loader, B. D., Hardey, M., and Keeble, L. (2008). Health informatics for older people: A review of ICT facilitated integrated care for older people. *International Journal of Social Welfare*, 17(1), 46–53.
Londonwide Local Medical Committees. (2008). Polyclinics and your practice. https://www.lmc.org.uk/article.php?group_id=684&start=521&end=530
Loopstra, R., McKee, M., Katikireddi, S. V., Taylor-Robinson, D., Barr, B., and Stuckler, D. (2016). Austerity and old-age mortality in England: A longitudinal cross-local area analysis, 2007–2013. *Journal of the Royal Society of Medicine*, 109(3), 109–116.
LSE News. (2011). Doubling expenditure on the NHS between 1997 and 2010 had a variable impact on health system performance. http://www.lse.ac.uk/website-archive/newsAndMedia/newsArchives/2011/03/NHSreport.aspx
Lyotard, J. F. (1984). *The Postmodern Condition*. University of Minnesota Press, Minneapolis.
Marcuse, H. (1969). *An Essay on Liberation*. Beacon Press, Boston.

Marmot, M. (2017). UCL IHE analysis of Eurostat life expectancy data. http://www.instituteofhealthequity.org/in-the-news/news-coverage/ucl-ihe-analysis-of-eurostat-life-expectancy-data---comment-piece

Maskovsky, J. (2000). "Managing" the poor: Neoliberalism, Medicaid HMOs and the triumph of consumerism among the poor. *Medical Anthropology*, 19(2), 121–146.

McCafferty, P. (1994). *Living Independently: A Study of the Housing Needs of Elderly and Disabled People*. HMSO, for the Department of the Environment, London.

McGrath, K. (2005). Doing critical research in information systems: A case of theory and practice not informing each other. *Information Systems Journal*, 15(2), 85–101.

MedAnth/Medical Anthropology Wiki. (2010). http://medanth.wikispaces.com/Governmentality

Miller, P., and Rose, N. (2008). *Governing the Present: Administering Social and Personal Life*. Polity, Cambridge.

Minkler, M. (1991). Gold in gray: Reflections on business' discovery of the elderly market. In M. Minkler and C. L. Estes (eds.), *Critical Perspectives on Aging: The Political and Moral Economy of Growing Old*, pp. 81–93. Baywood, New York.

Miskelly, F. G. (2001). Assistive technology in elderly care. *Age and Ageing*, 30, 455–458.

Mitev, N. N. (2005). Are social constructivist approaches critical?: The case of IS failure. In D. Howcroft and E. M. Trauth (eds.), *Handbook of Critical Information Systems Research: Theory and Application*, pp. 70–103. Edward Elgar, Cheltenham.

Mol, A. (2008). *The Logic of Care: Health and the Problem of Patient Choice*. Routledge, London.

Moody, H. R. (1992). *Ethics in an Aging Society*. Johns Hopkins University Press, Baltimore.

Mort, M., Roberts, C., and Callen, B. (2013). Ageing with telecare: Care or coercion in austerity? *Sociology of Health & Illness*, 35(6), 799–812.

National Archives. (2010). Whole system demonstrators. http://webarchive.nationalarchives.gov.uk/+/www.dh.gov.uk/en/Healthcare/longtermconditions/wholesystemdemonstrators/index.htm

National Archives. (2016). Royal commission on long term care for the Elderly: Registered files. http://discovery.nationalarchives.gov.uk/details/r/C14968

National Archives. (2017). Accessible publications. http://www.nationalarchives.gov.uk/information-management/producing-official-publications/publishing-guidance/accessible-publications/

NCPOP / National Centre for the Protection of Older People. (2009). Constructing ageing and age identities: A case study of newspaper discourses. https://pdfs.semanticscholar.org/8386/89c432ffa72011f90aa0a7f97fca94ecd333.pdf

NHS Executive – Department of Health. (1998). *Information for Health: An Information Strategy for the Modern NHS 1998–2005*. London.

NHS Providers. (2018). The NHS provider sector. http://nhsproviders.org/topics/delivery-and-performance/the-nhs-provider-sector

NICE. (2013). Falls in older people: Assessing risk and prevention https://www.nice.org.uk/guidance/CG161/chapter/introduction#populations-covered-by-this-guideline

Nonhoff, M. (2017). Discourse analysis as critique. *Palgrave Communications*, 3, 17074.

O'Farrell, C. (2005). *Michel Foucault*. SAGE, London.

O'Farrell, C. (2007). Key concepts – Michel Foucault. http://www.michel-foucault.com/concepts/

Olssen, M. (2014). Discourse, complexity, normativity: Tracing the elaboration of Foucault's materialist concept of discourse. *Open Review of Educational Research*, 1(1), 28–55.

ONS / Office for National Statistics. (2013). Total household wealth by region and age group. http://webarchive.nationalarchives.gov.uk/20160109093919/http://www.ons.gov.uk/ons/rel/regional-trends/regional-economic-analysis/wealth-by-age-group-and-region--june-2013/rep-total-household-wealth-by-region-and-age-group.html

OpenDemocracy.(2014).Theonly'parity'formentalhealthisthatitisbeingcutand privatised as well. https://www.opendemocracy.net/ournhs/peter-beresford/only-parity-for-mental-health-is-that-it-is-being-cut-and-privatised-as-well

Oudshoorn, N. (2011). *Telecare Technologies and the Transformation of Healthcare*. Palgrave Macmillan, Basingstoke.

Papworth Trust. (2016). Disability in the United Kingdom - 2016: Facts and figures. https://equalityhub.org/wp-content/uploads/2018/02/Disability-Facts-and-Figures-2016.pdf

Patel, N. (1990). *A Race against Time*. Runnymede Trust, London.

Peszynski, K. J., and Corbitt, B. J. (2006). Politics, complexity, and systems implementation: Critically exposing power. *Social Science Computer Review*, 24(3), 326–341.

Phillipson, C. (1993). The sociology of retirement. In J. Bond, P. Coleman, and S. Peace (eds.), *Ageing and Society: An Introduction to Social Gerontology*, pp. 180–199. Sage, London.

Phillipson, C. (1998). *Reconstructing Old Age*. Sage Publications, London.

Phillipson, C., and Biggs, S. (1998). Modernity and identity: Themes and perspectives in the study of older adults. *Journal of Aging and Identity*, 3, 11.

Physicians for a National Health Program. (2007). Private finance initiative costs British NHS billions. http://www.pnhp.org/news/2007/september/private_finance_init.php

Potter, J. (1996). *Representing Reality. Discourse, Rhetoric and Social Construction*. SAGE, London.

Potter, J., and Wetherell, M. (1987). *Discourse and Social Psychology: Beyond Attitudes and Behaviour*. SAGE, London.

Powell, J., and Biggs, S. (2000). Managing old age: The disciplinary web of power, surveillance and normalization. *Journal of Aging and Identity*, 5(1), 3–13.

Powell, J. L., and Biggs, S. (2003). Foucauldian gerontology: A methodology for understanding aging. *Electronic Journal of Sociology*, 7(2), 1–14.

Powell, J. L., and Biggs, S. (2004). Ageing, technologies of self and biomedicine: A Foucauldian excursion. *International Journal of Sociology and Social Policy*, 24(6), 17–29.

Pozzebon, M. (2004). Conducting and evaluating critical interpretive research: Examining criteria as a key component in building a research tradition. In B. Kaplan, D. P. Truex, D. Wastell, A. T. Wood-Harper, and J. I. DeGross (eds.), *Information Systems Research: Relevant Theory and Informed Practice*, pp. 275–292. Kluwer Academic Publishers, Norwell, MA.

Rabinow, P. (1984). *The Foucault Reader*, vol. 1. Pantheon Books, New York.

Rabinow, P. (1996). *Essays on the Anthropology of Reason*. Princeton University Press, Princeton.

Reuters UK. (2017). Conservatives aim to end budget deficit by mid-2020s. https://uk.reuters.com/article/uk-britain-election-budget/conservatives-aim-to-end-budget-deficit-by-mid-2020s-idUKKCN18E1CO

Richardson, H. (2003). CRM in cll centres: The logic of practice. In M. Korpela, R. Montealegre, and A. Poulymenakou (eds.), *Organizational Information Systems in the Context of Globalization*, pp. 69–84. Kluwer Academic Publishers, Boston.

Richardson, H., Tapia, A., and Kvasny, L. (2006). Introduction: Applying critical theory to the study of ICT. *Social Science Computer Review*, 24(3), 1–8.

Riley, P. (1988). The ethnography of autonomy. In A. Brookes and P. Grundy (eds.), *Individualization and Autonomy in Language Learning*, pp. 12–34. Modern English Publications/ The British Council, London.

Roberts, J. (2013). UKHCA dementia strategy and plan – February 2013. https://www.ukhca.co.uk/pdfs/UKHCADementiaStrategy201202final.pdf

Roehr, B. (2013). Telehealth can be beneficial when used properly, say experts. *BMJ*, 346: f1995.

Rose, G. (2001). *Visual Methodologies: An Introduction to the Interpretation of Visual Materials*. SAGE, London

Rose, N. (1999). *Powers of Freedom: Reframing Political Thought*. Cambridge University Press, Cambridge.

Rose, N. (2001). The politics of life itself. *Theory, Culture and Society*, 18(6), 1–30.

Rose, N., and Novas, C. (2005). Biological citizenship. In A. Ong and S. Collier (eds.), *Global Assemblages: Technology, Politics and Ethics as Anthropological Problems*, pp. 439–463. Blackwell, Malden.

Royal Commission on Long Term Care. (1999). With respect to old age: Long term care - rights and responsibilities. The Stationery Office, London.

Sanders, C., Rogers, A., Bowen, R., Bower, P., Hirani, S., Cartwright, M., Fitzpatrick, R., Knapp, M., Barlow, J., Hendy, J., Chrysanthaki, T., Bardsley, M., and Newman, S. P. (2012). Exploring barriers to participation and

adoption of telehealth and telecare within the Whole System Demonstrator trial: A qualitative study. *BMC Health Services Research*, 12, 220.
Schermer, M. (2009). Telecare and self-management: Opportunity to change the paradigm? *Journal of Medical Ethics*, 35(11), 688–691.
Scottish Parliament. (2013). Consultation on proposal to abolish NHS prescription charges. http://www.parliament.scot/S2_MembersBills/Draft%20proposals/colinFoxNHSBill.pdf
Scott-Samuel, A., Bambra, C., Collins, C., Hunter, D. J., McCartney, G., and Smith, K. (2014). Neoliberalism in health care: The impact of Thatcherism on health and well-being in Britain. *International Journal of Health Services*, 44(1), 53–71.
Secretary of State for Health. (2000). The NHS plan. A plan for investment. A plan for reform. A Summary. http://www.nhshistory.net/nhsplan.pdf
Shaw, E. (2010). Privatization by stealth? The Blair government and public-private partnerships in the National Health Service. *Contemporary Politics*, 9(3), 277–292.
Sheyholislami, J. (2001). Critical discourse analysis. http://www.carleton.ca/~jsheyhol/cda.htm
Silva, L. (2005). Theoretical approaches for researching power and information systems: A Machiavellian view. In D. Howcroft and E. M. Trauth (eds.), *Handbook of Critical Information Systems Research: Theory and Application*, pp. 47–69. Edward Elgar, Cheltenham.
Sixsmith, A., and Sixsmith, J. (2008). Ageing in place in the United Kingdom. *Ageing International*, 32, 219–235.
Slater, G. (1930). *Poverty and the State*. Constable, London.
Smart, B. (1985). *Michel Foucault*. Routledge, London.
Sorell, T., and Draper, H. (2012). Telecare, surveillance, and the welfare state. *The American Journal of Bioethics: AJOB*, 12(9), 36–44.
Steventon, A., Bardsley, M., Billings, J., Dixon, J., Doll, H., Beynon, M, Hirani, S., Cartwright, M., Rixon, L., Knapp, M., Henderson, C., Rogers, A., Hendy J., Fitzpatrick, R., and Newman, S. (2013). Effect of telecare on use of health and social care services: Findings from the Whole Systems Demonstrator cluster randomised trial. *Age and Ageing*, 42(4), 501–508.
Steventon, A., Bardsley, M., Billings, J., Dixon, J., Doll, H., Hirani, S., Cartwright, M., Rixon, L., Knapp, M., Henderson, C., Rogers, A., Fitzpatrick, R., Hendy, J., and Newman, S. (2012). Effect of telehealth on use of secondary care and mortality: Findings from the Whole System Demonstrator cluster randomised trial. *BMJ*, 344, e3874.
Strehler, B. (1962). *Time, Cells and Aging*. Academic Press, New York.
TSA / Telecare Services Association. (2017a). About TSA. https://www.tsa-voice.org.uk/about-tsa
TSA. (2017b). Who endorses QSF? Retrieved November 5, 2017 from https://www.tsa-voice.org.uk/who-endorses-qsf
TSA. (2018). Nationwide survey of telecare use by local authorities. https://www.tsa-voice.org.uk/news_and_views/tsa-news/nationwide-survey-of-telecare-use-by-local-authorities/

Tunstall. (2018). Lancashire county council – Telecare at scale. https://www.tunstall.co.uk/resources/case-studies/2018/09/lancashire-county-council---telecare/
UK Housing. (2007). Innovation and good practice programme launched. http://www.uk-housing.co.uk/HMD/ARCHIVE/06/09/493/
UK Parliament. (2016). NHS professionals limited: Written statement - HLWS265. https://www.parliament.uk/business/publications/written-questions-answers-statements/written-statement/Lords/2016-11-17/HLWS265/
van Dijk, T. A. (2001). Critical discourse analysis. In D. Tannen, D. Schiffrin, and H. Hamilton (eds.), *Handbook of Discourse Analysis*, pp. 352–371. Blackwell, Oxford.
Wahlberg, A., and Rose, N. (2015). The governmentalization of living: Calculating global health. *Economy and Society*, 44(1), 60–90.
Wakefield, A., and Fleming, J. (2009). *The Sage Dictionary of Policing*. SAGE Publications, Los Angeles.
Walsh, B., and Gillett, G. (2011). Is evidence-based Medicine positivist? *The International Journal of Person Centered Medicine*, 1(2), 323–329.
Walsham, G. (2001). *Making a World of Difference: IT in a Global Context*. Wiley, Chichester.
Warnes, A. (1996). *Human Ageing and Later Life*. Edward Arnold, London.
Watt, N. (2000). Blair's £12bn pledge to NHS. https://www.theguardian.com/society/2000/jan/17/futureofthenhs.health1
Weedon, C. (2004). *Identity and Culture: Narratives of Difference and Belonging*. Open University Press, Berkshire.
Willcocks, L. P. (2004). Foucault, power/knowledge and information systems: Reconstructing the present. In J. Mingers and L. P. Willcocks (eds.), *Social Theory and Philosophy for Information Systems*, pp. 238–296. Wiley, Chichester.
Willcocks, L. P. (2006). Michel Foucault in the social study of ICTs: Critique and reappraisal. *Social Science Computer Review*, 24(3), 274–295.
Women's Budget Group. (2016). AFS 2016: Women's Budget Group response. https://wbg.org.uk/wp-content/uploads/2016/12/AFS2016_WBGreport_13Dec_final2.pdf
Yusif, S., Soar, J., and Hafeez-Baig, A. (2016). Older people, assistive technologies, and the barriers to adoption: A systematic review. *International Journal of Medical Informatics*, 94, 112–116.
Zuboff, S. (1988). *In the Age of the Smart Machine: The Future of Work and Power*. Basic Books, New York.

Appendices

Appendix A: References of all documents analysed

References

a) Health and social care publications of Government, Department of Health, and industry bodies, etc.

1. Anchor Trust. (1999). Using Telecare: The Experiences and Expectations of Older People.
2. Centre for Policy on Ageing. (2014). The Potential Impact of New Technologies, (July), 1–74. http://www.ageuk.org.uk/professionals/knowledge-hub-evidence-statistics/evidence-reviews/cpa-review-of-social-care/
3. Communities and Local Government Committee. (2017). Adult Social Care: Ninth Report of Session 2016–2017. House of Commons. https://www.publications.parliament.uk/pa/cm201617/cmselect/cmcomloc/1103/1103.pdf
4. CSIP / Care Services Improvement Partnership. (2005). Telecare Implementation Guide. https://www.housinglin.org.uk/Topics/type/Telecare-Implementation-Guide-July-2005-/
5. Department of Health. (1998). Modernising Social Services [The National Archives]. London.
6. Department of Health. (2005a). Strategic Business Case Models for Telecare, (July).
7. Department of Health. (2005b). Building Telecare in England.
8. Department of Health. (2005c). Independence, Well-being and Choice.
9. Department of Health. (2006). Our Health, Our Care, Our Say: A New Direction for Community Services. The Stationery Office.
10. Department of Health. (2009). Whole Systems Demonstrators: An Overview of Telecare and Telehealth. London. http://www.housingcare.org/information/detail-2578-quality-choice-for-older-peoples-housing-strategic-fram.aspx

11 Department of Health. (2010a). A Vision for Adult Social Care. https://www.gov.uk/government/publications/lac-dh-2010-7-the-vision-for-adult-social-care-and-supporting-documents
12 Department of Health. (2010b). Prioritising Need in the Context of Putting People First: A Whole System Approach to Eligibility for Social Care – Guidance on Eligibility Criteria for Adult Social Care.
13 Department of Health. (2011a). Whole System Demonstrator Programme: Headline Findings. London.
14 Department of Health. (2011b). Health and Social Care Bill 2011.
15 Department of Health. (2012). A Concordat between the Department of Health and the Telehealth and Telecare Industry, 1–4.
16 Department of Health. (2012). Caring for Our Future: Some Ideas on How We Can Make Social Care Better.
17 Department of Health. (2014). The Care Act: Easy Read version, 5. https://www.gov.uk/government/uploads/system/uploads/attachment_data/file/365345/Making_Sure_the_Care_Act_Works_EASY_READ.pdf
18 Department of Health. (2015). NHS Constitution for England. https://www.gov.uk/government/publications/the-nhs-constitution-for-england
19 Department of Health. (2017). The Care Bill – Reforming What and How People Pay for their Care and Support.
20 Department of Health, & Care Quality Commission. (2017a). Adult Social Care: Quality Matters.
21 Department of Health, & Care Quality Commission. (2017b). Adult Social Care: Quality Matters – Easy Read Version.
22 Department of Health, & DETR. (2001a). Quality and Choice for Older People's Housing: A Strategic Framework (Summary).
23 Department of Health, & DETR. (2001b). Quality and Choice for Older People's Housing: A Strategic Framework. http://www.housingcare.org/information/detail-2578-quality-choice-for-older-peoples-housing-strategic-fram.aspx
24 Government Equalities Office. (2011). The Equality Act, Making Equality Real: Easy Read Document, 38. https://assets.publishing.service.gov.uk/government/uploads/system/uploads/attachment_data/file/85039/easy-read.pdf
25 HM Government. (2007). Putting People First: A Shared Vision and Commitment to the Transformation of Adult Social Care, 8. http://webarchive.nationalarchives.gov.uk/20130107105354/http:/www.dh.gov.uk/en/Publicationsandstatistics/Publications/PublicationsPolicyAndGuidance/DH_081118
26 HM Government. (2009). Shaping the Future of Care Together. http://www.cpa.org.uk/cpa/Shaping_future_of_care_together.pdf
27 HM Government. (2010). Building the National Care Service.
28 HM Government. (2012a). Caring for Our Future: Reforming Care and Support.

Appendices 131

29 HM Government. (2012b). Caring for Our Future: Reforming Care and Support (EasyRead version).
30 HM Government. (2015). 2010 to 2015 Government Policy: Long Term Health Conditions. https://www.gov.uk/government/publications/2010-to-2015-government-policy-long-term-health-conditions/2010-to-2015-government-policy-long-term-health-conditions
31 Jarrett, T. (2017). Social care: Government Reviews and Policy Proposals for Paying for Care since 1997 (England). House of Commons Library Briefing Papers.
32 King, J., Kohn, E., Lee, J., Lim, M., & Luczynska, M. (2010). Improving Service Delivery to an Ageing population: Strategies for UK Local Authorities (MPA Programme Capstone Report for Deloitte Consulting LLP). London.
33 NHS England. (2012). NHS Long Term Conditions Flyer. http://3millionlives.co.uk/wp-content/uploads/2012/11/3ML-telehealth-and-telecare-selfcare-leafelt-FINAL.pdf
34 NHS Executive. (2005). Information for Health: An Information Strategy for the Modern NHS 1998–2005.
35 Office of the Deputy Prime Minister. (2006). Local Authority Circular: Preventative Technology Grant 2006/07–2007/08.http://www.dh.gov.uk/prod_consum_dh/groups/dh_digitalassets/@dh/@en/documents/digitalasset/dh_4132169.pdf
36 Roberts, J. (2013). UKHCA Dementia Strategy and Plan, (3083104).
37 Secretary of State for Health. (2000). The NHS Plan: A Summary.
38 Secretary of State for Health. (2011). The NHS Plan.
39 TSA/Telecare Services Association. (2016a). Putting People First: Commissioning for Connected Care, Homes and Communities, (October).
40 TSA. (2016b). White Paper Launch 1-page summary, (October 2016).

b) Key texts whose forewords have been coded

1 Department of Health. (2005b). Building Telecare in England.
2 Department of Health. (2005c). Independence, Well-being and Choice.
3 Department of Health. (2006). Our Health, Our Care, Our Say: A New Direction for Community Services. The Stationery Office.
4 Department of Health, & DETR. (2001b). Quality and Choice for Older People's Housing: A Strategic Framework. http://www.housingcare.org/information/detail-2578-quality-choice-for-older-peoples-housing-strategic-fram.aspx
5 HM Government. (2009). Shaping the Future of Care Together. http://www.cpa.org.uk/cpa/Shaping_future_of_care_together.pdf
6 HM Government. (2010). Building the National Care Service.
7 Telecare Services Association. (2016a). Putting People First: Commissioning for Connected Care, Homes and Communities, (October).

c) Documents whose illustrations have been coded

Public sector images are licensed under the Open Government Licence for Public Sector Information v3.0- http://www.nationalarchives.gov.uk/doc/open-government-licence/version/3/

1. Department of Health. (2005). Strategic Business Case Models for Telecare, (July).
2. Department of Health. (2005b). Building Telecare in England.
3. Department of Health. (2006). Our Health, Our Care, Our Say: A New Direction for Community Services. The Stationery Office. https://www.gov.uk/government/uploads/system/uploads/attachment_data/file/272238/6737.pdf
4. Department of Health. (2009). Whole Systems Demonstrators: An Overview of Telecare and Telehealth. London. http://www.housingcare.org/information/detail-2578-quality-choice-for-older-peoples-housing-strategic-fram.aspx
5. Department of Health. (2010). Prioritising Need in the Context of Putting People First: A Whole System Approach to Eligibility for Social Care – Guidance on Eligibility Criteria for Adult Social Care, England 2010.
6. Department of Health. (2012). Caring for Our Future: Some Ideas on How We Can Make Social Care Better.
7. Department of Health, & Care Quality Commission. (2017a). Adult Social Care: Quality Matters.
8. Department of Health, & Care Quality Commission. (2017b). Adult Social Care: Quality Matters – Easy Read Version.
9. HM Government. (2009). Shaping the Future of Care Together. http://www.cpa.org.uk/cpa/Shaping_future_of_care_together.pdf
10. HM Government. (2010). Building the National Care Service.
11. HM Government. (2012a). Caring for Our Future: Reforming Care and Support.
12. HM Government. (2012b). Caring for Our Future: Reforming Care and Support (EasyRead version).
13. NHS England. (2012). NHS Long Term Conditions Flyer. http://3millionlives.co.uk/wp-content/uploads/2012/11/3ML-telehealth-and-telecare-selfcare-leafelt-FINAL.pdf

Appendix B: Visual Exhibits

Public sector images in this appendix are licensed under the Open Government Licence for Public Sector Information v3.0- http://www.nationalarchives.gov.uk/doc/open-government-licence/version/3/

Appendices 133

B.1 'The Balance of Care Model' in *Strategic Business Case Models for Telecare* (Department of Health, 2005a, p. 8)

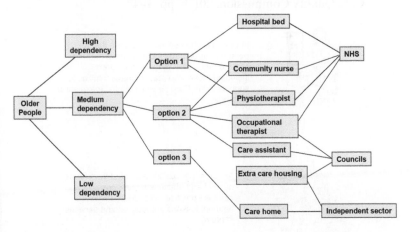

B.2 From *Adult Social Care: Quality Matters* (Department of Health and Care Quality Commission, 2017a, p. 10)

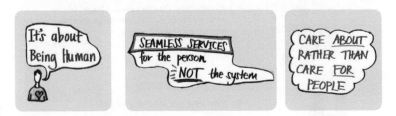

B.3 From *Adult Social Care: Quality Matters* (Department of Health and Care Quality Commission, 2017a, p. 8)

> By following these principles and encouraging others to do the same, we will promote high-quality, person-centred care, and support services to enable people using services to say:
> - "I feel in control and safe"
> - "I have the information I need when I need it"
> - "I have access to a range of support that helps me live my life"
> - "I am in control of my support, in my own way"
> - "I have considerate support delivered by competent staff"
> - "I can decide the kind of support I need"
>
> Source: Think Local Act Personal (TLAP)

134 *Appendices*

B.4 'What person-centred care looks like for people' in *Adult Social Care: Quality Matters–Easy Read version* (Department of Health & Care Quality Commission, 2017b, pp. 3–4)

For people who use services, care that is person-centred must focus on what matters most to them, their families and carers, including those who may not have families to support them. Care services should make sure that they:

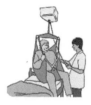

- Are safe: people are protected from harm, neglect and abuse wherever possible and can take positive risks. When mistakes happen, lessons are learned and services improve.

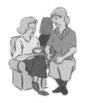

- Are effective: People's care is based on what we know is good, and helps them to enjoy a good quality of life.

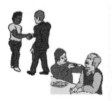

- Give people a positive experience by being:
    - caring: staff treat people with compassion, dignity and respect

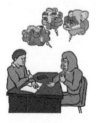

- responsive: services meet people's different needs and help them make as many decisions as possible about their own care and the way that care is planned for everyone.

B.5 'Putting People First approach' in *Prioritising Need in the Context of Putting People First: A Whole System Approach to Eligibility for Social Care* (Department of Health, 2010, p. 37)

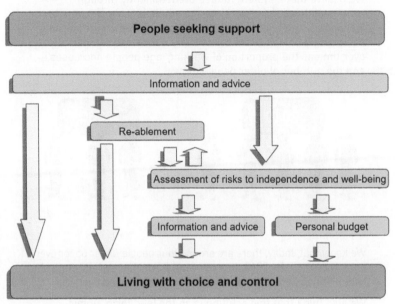

B.6 From *Building the National Care Service* (HM Government, 2010, p. 117)

"I feel the service user must be the person to decide what they get and how they choose to use it."

Public response to the Consultation

B.7 From *Building the National Care Service* (HM Government, 2010, pp. 127–128)

We believe that a system funded predominantly through increased taxation for working-age adults (such as income tax or National Insurance) would place a large burden on the working-age population – and this burden would increase significantly over time as the proportion of working-age people decreases, and the number of older people grows.

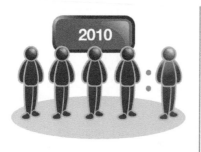
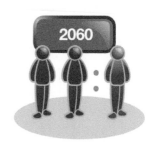

We know that, today, there are around four people under 65 for every person over 65. By 2060, this ratio will have changed dramatically, with just two people under 65 for every person aged over 65.

We also think that this solution is, in the long term, unfair between generations. The majority of people to benefit from a fully tax-funded system would be older people, and yet it is working-age adults who would face the largest burden in paying for it. We think that it is fairer to have a more targeted system to bring additional funding into the care and support system. We do appreciate that not all older people are well-off, but according to data from the Office for National Statistics, those aged between 65 and 74 are the second wealthiest age group in Britain, with an average total household wealth of £284,500, excluding private pension wealth. Those aged between 75 and 84 have an average of £235,000, excluding private pensions.[6] By contrast, many younger people have significant debts from mortgages or student loans.

B.8 From *Caring for Our Future: Reforming Care and Support (Easy Read version)* (HM Government, 2012b, p. 2)

Most importantly, we want to help people:

- to be more **independent**

- to have choice and control over their care and support

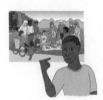

- to live their lives in the way they want

B.9 From *Caring for Our Future: Reforming Care and Support* (HM Government, 2012a, p. 28)

> ### Telecare supporting independence[32]
>
> Mr Montague was a 47-year-old man who had experienced serious epileptic fits over a long period of time. This affected his mental capacity, especially his short-term memory. His epilepsy was managed by medication but this left him drowsy. Following the installation of a telecare system, he felt enabled to move from shared supported housing to a single tenancy where he could live more independently. Unfortunately, Mr Montague had a bad accident, but he was wearing his falls alarm so the rapid response minimised the consequences of his fall.

B.10 From *Our Health, Our Care, Our Say: A New Direction for Community Services* (Department of Health, 2006, p. 62)

> **CASE STUDY**
>
> **Innovative GP services**
>
> The James Wigg Practice in Kentish Town – an inner-city London neighbourhood with high levels of disadvantage and health inequalities – is demonstrating the range of services that can be provided by primary care. The practice has GPs and nurses, of course, but it offers so much more.
>
> Visiting specialists include an alcohol counsellor, a drug counsellor, an adult psychologist and psychiatrist, an ophthalmologist and a rheumatologist. Clinics are run by practice nurses for many ongoing conditions, including diabetes, asthma, hypertension and quitting smoking.
>
> The practice makes extensive use of information techology. This means that patients can order repeat prescriptions using the internet. This emphasis on information technology has led to the practice being awarded beacon status. Patients can also conduct telephone consultations with doctors if they need advice or want to ascertain if they need to make an appointment.

B.11 From *Building Telecare in England* (Department of Health, 2005b, p. 9)

> **Case Study 1**
>
> Mrs A has dementia and was starting to forget to turn off the gas when cooking. She had a gas detector installed, with an automatic shut off valve when gas was detected in the air. This enabled Mrs A to stay in her own home, and still cook for herself.
>
> In time, a movement detector was added. It can differentiate between her opening the door to retrieve the milk delivery and when she opens the door and leaves the flat. Carers are not, therefore, alerted every time the door opens, but can intervene if appropriate and help if she leaves the house on her own.

B.12 From *Building Telecare in England* (Department of Health, 2005b, p. 9)

> **Case Study 2**
>
> Mrs B has a history of falling. Following discharge from hospital she was provided with a basic telecare package that included a bed pressure sensor that could detect when she left the bed during the night and turned on the lighting to her bathroom. It would then trigger an alarm if she did not return to bed within an agreed time.
>
> The package was programmed to record how many times Mrs B left her bed during the night. A few weeks after it was installed it was noticed at the control centre that Mrs B's nocturnal visits to the bathroom had increased significantly over a three day period. They alerted a care professional and Mrs B was diagnosed with a urinary tract infection which was then quickly treated enabling a full and quick recovery.

B.13 From *Building Telecare in England* (Department of Health, 2005b, p. 11)

> **Case Study 3: Telecare supporting people with dementia**
>
> One project aims to support the independence of people with dementia by using technology to compensate for disabilities arising from dementia.
>
> Referrals to the project can be made by a social or health care professional, and a full assessment is undertaken, to identify technology tailored to meet specific needs. The project worker also has responsibility for obtaining and arranging for the installation of this technology, and liaising with the local control centre who co-ordinate any social response.
>
> Risk management is a major feature of the project, for example, technology that can detect the presence of gas and isolate the supply to a stove or fire that may have been left on unlit, and an alert can be raised. This means people with dementia can continue to cook their own meals.
>
> Key findings were that people without telecare were four times more likely to leave the community for hospital or residential care over the 21 month evaluation period. The equivalent cost saving was £1.5 million over the 21 months.

B.14 From *Building Telecare in England* (Department of Health, 2005b, p. 11)

> **Case Study 4: Telecare to support people with Long Term Conditions**
>
> This project is part of the overall Long Term Conditions strategy and part of the local assistive technology programme, a joint health and social care initiative. The service which is a health project is situated in the council alarm service and is co-ordinated by a nurse based in the call centre. The project aims to help individuals with long term conditions to:
>
> - Self manage and increase treatment/medication compliance.
> - Identify earlier than currently possible when patients' conditions deteriorate, thus averting an acute exacerbation of their condition.
> - Increase access to, and amount of, information readily available to healthcare professionals.
> - Reduce the risk of individuals on the project becoming 'Intensive Service Users'.
>
> 25 'suites of equipment' are available and are being used for as many people as possible over the first year. People will be on the service for 30–60 days in order that they becoming self-managing.

B.15 From *Building Telecare in England* (Department of Health, 2005b, p. 12)

> **Case Study 5: Telecare to support vulnerable adults**
>
> This project has an emphasis on using technology to improve the lives of the most vulnerable in society. The council has taken a flexible approach so that health and social care professionals can refer people to the project. To be eligible, the case has to meet one of a number of national objectives e.g. falls prevention, supporting carers, keeping people in their own homes for longer, and preventing delayed discharges. The project initially began in one area, but is now being rolled out to the rest of the borough.

Appendices 141

B.16 From *Building Telecare in England* (Department of Health, 2005b, p. 12)

> **Case Study 6: Telecare as part of Intermediate Care**
>
> A number of authorities use telecare as part of their intermediate care service. On discharge from hospital people's homes are fitted with a basic telecare package. They also receive regular visits and calls from the community alarm service alongside rehabilitation and care from health and social care staff. The telecare equipment and service are provided free of charge for six weeks. It is a very popular part of the package and one which many individuals choose to retain.

B.17 From *Shaping the Future of Care Together* (HM Government 2009, p. 52).

> **Case study: Re-ablement and telecare**
>
> After he had a stroke, Terence was at risk of falling and was not able to be at home safely on his own. Because he wanted to leave hospital, he was discharged two weeks early to a special flat with additional support. While he was there he received rehabilitation from the intermediate care team, but also built up his confidence to live independently and had a falls detector, bed sensor and gas detector. He returned to his own flat several weeks later and did not require further care.

B.18 From *Whole Systems Demonstrators: An Overview of Telecare and Telehealth* (Department of Health, 2009, p. 21)

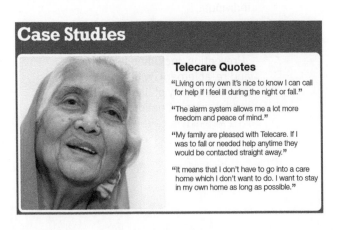

Case Studies

Telecare Quotes

"Living on my own it's nice to know I can call for help if I feel ill during the night or fall."

"The alarm system allows me a lot more freedom and peace of mind."

"My family are pleased with Telecare. If I was to fall or needed help anytime they would be contacted straight away."

"It means that I don't have to go into a care home which I don't want to do. I want to stay in my own home as long as possible."

B.19 From *Building the National Care Service* (HM Government, 2010, p. 50)

> **Telecare in Newham[19]**
>
> Ex-nurse Jill, 77 years old, is registered blind and has a frail physique from childhood polio. As a result, she is prone to falls. Though she has a carer who comes twice a week to help her around the home, a concern for her is being at home alone if she has an accident with nobody there to help her. In 2008, she had two falls at home, which prompted her to seek an alternative solution.
>
> Jill now has a pendant she can press if she needs assistance, a heat detector in the kitchen to warn of high temperatures, and a radio pull cord in the bathroom.
>
> She said, "Because of my nursing experience I was thrilled to hear these things were being developed to help protect vulnerable people and help them maintain their dignity so they can feel like they are still capable of carrying on themselves. Now I can have a bath on my own. I feel safer and it helps me to retain my independence."

B.20 From *Building the National Care Service* (HM Government, 2010, p. 90)

> "All care should be person centred and specific to the individual."
> Public response to the Consultation

> "Prevention, including telecare and re-ablement, will help to improve quality of life and will reduce support needs."
> Public response to the Consultation

Appendices 143

B.21 'Types of Resources and Services' in *Prioritising Need in the Context of Putting People First: A Whole System Approach to Eligibility for Social Care* (Department of Health, 2010, p. 17)

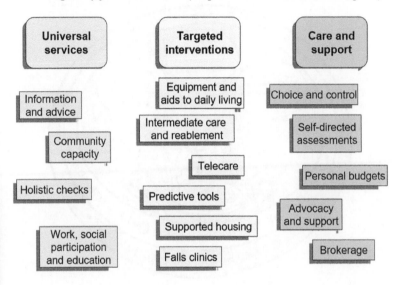

B.22 From *NHS Long Term Conditions Flyer* (NHS England, 2012, p. 1)

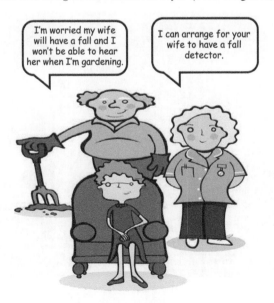

144 *Appendices*

B.23 From *Adult Social Care: Quality Matters* (Department of Health and Care Quality Commission, 2017a, p. 5)

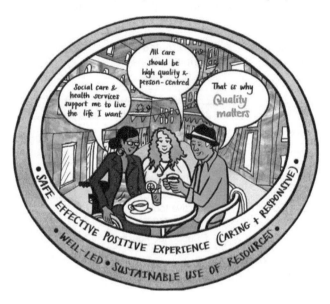

B.24 From *Building the National Care Service* (HM Government, 2010, p. 76)

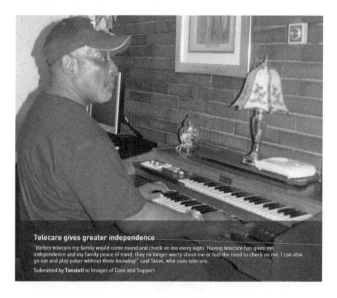

B.25 'Empowering and enabling individuals to take control' in *Our Health, Our Care, Our Say: A New Direction for Community Services* (Department of Health, 2006, p. 111)

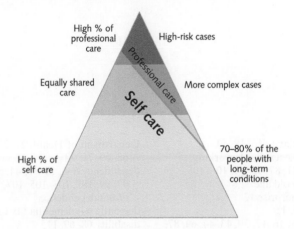

Index

active ageing 6, 15, 18, 53
age: middle age 8, 11; working age 6, 71, 87, 92, 99, 106–108; *see also* old age
ageing enterprise 12
ageism 13, 15
assessment 16–17, 39, 43–44, 69, 87, 96, 97, 101–102
austerity 61–62, 64, 106

Biggs, S. 14–16, 27–28, 39, 96
bio-power 49–51, 73, 75

care: caps 62–63, 92, 96; cost of 22, 24, 65, 69, 93, 96, 108; management (*see* managerialism in care); means test 62–63, 93, 96; research 23–25; technologies 3, 28, 65, 76, 94
Care Standards Act 66
choice 17, 25, 42, 61, 65, 78–79, 86, 87, 95, 97, 104–105
community alarm 19, 66, 68
Conservative government 59–63; *see also* Thatcher government
consumerism 65, 79, 80, 86, 101; consumer culture 2, 14; consumerist view of old age 12; gold in grey 1, 14
continuity *see* discontinuity
council *see* local authority
critical discourse analysis 35, 58, 75, 85
critical theory 29–33, 39

Department of Health 21–22, 25, 59, 68–69, 71–72
dependency 5–6, 14–16, 44, 53, 95, 97, 99, 101, 103–105, 107, 108; *see also* independence
dementia 64; dementia tax 63
disability 68–69, 115
discontinuity 38, 40–41
discourse 32, 37, 36, 55, 107; contradictory coexisting discourses 14, 108, 115; discursive level 34–35; of decline 14–15; of old age 2, 14, 54, 88, 100–109, 103, 108; *see also* critical discourse analysis; old age
distributive justice 27, 105, 106, 108
dividing practices 47–49, 55, 74, 88, 90, 92

emancipation 30–31, 53
embodied practices 10
empowerment 16–17, 27, 33, 39, 101, 104–105
episteme 40, 47, 57
Estes, C. 9, 12, 94

Fairclough, N. 35–36, 75
Featherstone, M. 11, 14
Feenberg, A. 32
Foucauldian discourse analysis 37, 58
Foucault, M. 3, 12, 14, 17, 29, 33, 37–45, 52, 97, 100–101; *The History of Sexuality* 12, 48; *The Order of Discourse* 36; *The Order of Things* 47; *The Subject and Power* 44, 47
Frankfurt School 29–31, 33, 41

Index   147

gender: differences in life course 6; inequality 11, 64
genealogy 39–42, 115
gerontology 9, 12, 47; critical 2, 12–13; Foucauldian 13–14, 27
Giddens, A. 10, 31
governmentalisation 37, 49, 51–52, 55, 73, 107–108
governmentality *see* governmentalisation
grand discourses 55; of old age 2–3, 15, 17–18, 101–108, 112

Habermas, J. 29–31
Hacking, I. 45–46, 73
Hepworth, M. 11, 14
hollow state 9, 53, 57, 94, 96, 99, 101
human kind 42, 45–46, 55, 73, 89, 109

identity: definition 42–46, 48, 52, 55, 74, 106; of old age 3, 8, 44–45, 49, 56, 87–88, 100, 106–107, 115
independence 18, 65, 73, 79, 85, 94, 96–97, 103–105, 108
individualisation 10–13, 49, 52, 98, 101, 108
inequality (economic) 64, 92, 106, 109, 111, 114
information systems (IS): critical research of 30–34; telecare information systems 29, 54, 115
intergenerational contract 83, 92, 98–99, 101

Klecun, E. 32, 95

Labour government 58–60; *see also* New Labour
lifestyle 6, 10, 53, 94, 99, 102
Linkins, K. 9
local authority 23, 60–64, 93–97
localism 73, 81, 94, 101
looping effects 45–47, 74, 109, 115

managerialism in care 16–17, 86, 96, 99, 105, 112
Marcuse, H. 30

marketisation 7, 61, 97, 101
medical gaze 8, 56
modernisation of services 65–66, 73, 77, 79, 84, 93, 94
modernity 10, 56, 98; first (simple) modernity 6; late modernity (*see* postmodernism); pre-modernity 10; reflexive modernity 11; *see also* postmodernism
modes of objectification 3, 29, 47, 74, 115
Moody, H.R. 12
morality 28, 100; moral framework 6, 53

neoliberalism 16, 52, 97
New Labour 60–61, 109
NHS (National Health Service), history of 53, 58–65
NICE (National Institute for Health and Care Excellence) 20
normalisation 34, 39, 50–53, 55, 90, 105, 112

old age: definition 55; discourses of (*see* discourse); grand discourses of (*see* grand discourses); history of in Britain 5–17; identity of (*see* identity); medicalisation of 2, 14, 101; problematisation of as a social issue 1, 5, 13, 85, 93, 99, 101, 112; as a separate group 1, 11–14, 44, 53–54, 77, 88, 91–92, 106–107; *see also* discourse; identity; pension

panopticon 33, 50, 56
pension *see* state pension
Phillipson, C. 11, 98–99
policy recommendations 114
politics of participation 16, 96, 108
postmodernism 9, 11–13, 53, 56, 98–99; postmodern life course 2; postmodernist approaches in research 30–33
Powell, J. 15–16, 27–28
power 36, 41–42, 45, 50, 55; sovereign 37, 55, 75
power/knowledge 37–38, 49–50, 52, 55, 73

Index

Preventative Technology Grant 21, 68, 70
privatisation of services 9, 52, 59–61, 79, 94, 100

randomised control trial 22, 24, 32, 71, 91
regime of truth 33, 45, 57, 107
responsibilisation 26, 95, 99, 101
retirement 1, 6–9, 11, 53
Rose, N. 25, 52

Schermer, M. 27, 104–105
scientific classification 47–49, 55, 74, 88, 90–92
social care *see* care
social inclusion 6–7, 16, 66, 96
social responsibility 13, 77, 83–88, 93, 97–100, 105, 108, 114
social work 15, 18, 102
sociology of ageing 9
state pension 1, 5, 8–9
Steventon, A. 22, 24
subjectification 14, 44–45, 100; self-subjectification 47–48, 73, 115
subjectivity *see* identity
surveillance 26–27, 91, 104, 108

technology: critical theory of 32; as an electronic panopticon 33; un-neutrality 33
technologies of the self 48–49, 74, 109
telecare: cycle 20; history 18–23; initiatives and trials 2, 21–23, 66–67, 71–72; provision (*see* local authority); technologies 2, 18, 21, 68, 112, 115; *see also* information systems
Telecare Services Association (TSA) 76, 94, 110
telehealth 21–22, 25, 32
Thatcher government 1, 7–8, 59
thematisation: absent theme 36, 85–86; of policies 72, 77–89
3ML (3millionlives) 22, 25

Weedon, C. 43, 106
welfare 13, 15–16, 18, 52, 96–97, 102–108; funding crisis of 1, 54, 59; reforms 7, 66; state 1, 5–13, 26, 46, 53, 59, 95–98, 108
Whole System Demonstrators (WSD) 22, 24, 71–72, 91
Willcocks, L. 33
Wodak, R. 36